The Yoga of
the Nine Emotions

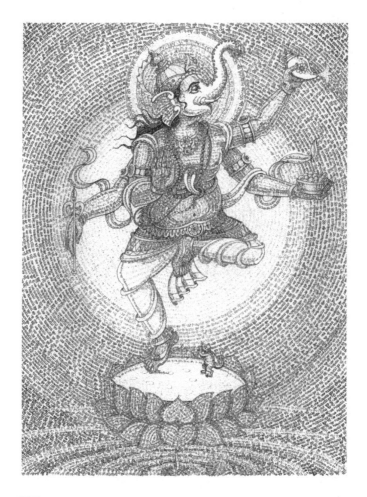

aum
Gajananam bhootganadhisevitam
kapitthya jamboo phalasaara bhakshakam
Umasutam shokvinashkarakam
namami Vighneshwar padpankajam
aum

Elephant-faced, worshipped by all existing beings,
tasting the elephant apple (kaith) *and jamun fruit* (jambolana),
the son of Uma, destroyer of grief,
I bow to the lotus feet of Ganesha, who is Lord of all.

The Yoga of the Nine Emotions

THE TANTRIC PRACTICE OF RASA SADHANA

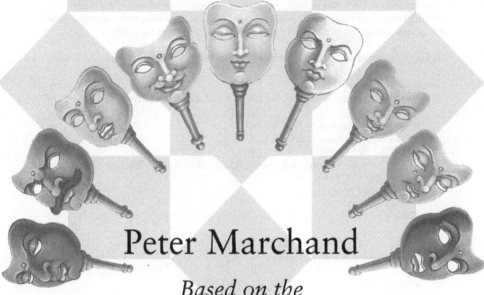

Peter Marchand

Based on the
Teachings of Harish Johari

Destiny Books
Rochester, Vermont

Destiny Books
One Park Street
Rochester, Vermont 05767, USA
www.DestinyBooks.com

Destiny Books is a division of Inner Traditions International

LIBRARY OF CONGRESS CATALOGING-IN-PUBLICATION DATA

Marchand, Peter, 1963–
    The yoga of the nine emotions : the tantric practice of rasa sadhana / Peter Marchand.
        p. cm.
    "Based on the teachings of Harish Johari."
    Includes bibliographical references and index.
    ISBN 978-1-59477-094-4
    1. Yoga. 2. Rasas. 3. Tantrism. 4. Johari, Harish, 1934–1999—Teachings. I. Johari, Harish, 1934–1999. II. Title.
    B132.Y6M299 2006
    294.5'436—dc22

                                                                        2006002970

Printed and bound in the United States

10   9   8   7   6

Text design and layout by Virginia Scott Bowman
This book was typeset in Sabon and Avenir with Nuptial Script and Avenir as the display typefaces

To send correspondence to the author of this book, mail a first-class letter to the author c/o Inner Traditions • Bear & Company, One Park Street, Rochester, VT 05767, and we will forward the communication.

Contents

Part Three: Working with Our Rasas

Part Four: Our Rasas in Society

Acknowledgments

I owe all credit for this book to Sri Harish Johari, who gave the "Rasa Siddhanta" lecture series that forms the principal basis of this book. All credit goes to him not only because the content is thus really his, but also because I could not have written it without his contribution to my personal development as my teacher since 1983.

As Harish Johari left his body in August 1999 without having written a book on the Rasas, the essences of our emotions, he left me with a great challenge and opportunity. The writing of this book has offered me more in terms of personal growth than the material could ever have given me in any other way. I can only feel very grateful to him.

The Rasas lectures by Harish Johari took place in 1997 in Belgium and were spread out over a period of nine days, for a total of about twenty hours of actual lectures. In between, the small group of students from Belgium and the Netherlands would cook and paint and talk and more, working with the teachings of Harish Johari in a most unique way. And of course, there was no escape from confronting our emotions during that time. This was especially true because Harish Johari, as a real elder brother or Dada, was tickling and teasing us to reveal them and face them. All the while he remained the teacher of many ancient ways, which each student could choose from according to his or her desire and temperament.

I also thank Marian Duys for freely offering her house as the wonderful home where Harish Johari's lectures in Belgium took place, that year and many years before that. While having to act out the role of the hostess to all those visitors, she still found the time to dutifully record every minute of the lectures on tape. My own notes represented only a fraction of the richness of the teaching, so I could have done nothing without her.

I thank the Johari family that allowed me to convert the content of the tapes into a book and to interpret this teaching in my own way. I hope that they still find enough of the original spirit within, in spite of my attempt to also look at the Rasas from a Western point of view. I thank Christine Grünwald for typing out the majority of the lecture tapes. I thank Pieter Weltevrede for creating the great cover image of the Rasas and the image of Ganesha for the frontispiece. I thank those at the publisher Destiny Books for being a constant source of good advice and enthusiasm from the very moment they knew about this project. And I thank the following friends and family for reading through the draft version of this book and providing me with so many interesting comments: André Marchand, Chris Marchand, Christine Grünwald, Dominique Van Gerven, Geva Weltevrede, Heidi Rauhut, James Daley, Joe Baxter, John Marchand, Mme. Champagne, Mohit Johri, Monique Marchand, Narmada Devi, Nelleke Sparling, Pieter Weltevrede, Rudy Kuhn, and Wil Geraets. Special thanks also are due for the moral support by Christina Richã Devi.

I thank the Indian people of so many generations for passing on this ancient knowledge, up to the point where my teacher learned it from his parents and his teachers. One does not often think about Indian people as being stubborn, but they are very stubborn at preserving good things.

Of course, I thank everybody that contributed to my life and provided me with the practical experience necessary to understand the play of Rasas and to train my emotional control with Rasa Sadhana, among which of course my parents, family, and son are of foremost importance, along with some of my dear friends and a few of my dear enemies.

Last—but by far the most worthy of gratitude—is the divine Mother on whose body we are all allowed to enjoy this game of Rasas. In these times, in which the imagination is rather limited when it comes to being grateful, I simply thank life.

Note on the Use of Sanskrit Terms

Converting the Sanskrit language to English is difficult because its alphabet has many more characters. It is particularly difficult to convert the Sanskrit characters that combine vowels and consonants to English without creating spellings that appear strange to some Indian readers. For example, the word "Rasa" is actually written "Ras" in Sanskrit, and a short sounding final "a" is implied. We have included such vowels to come as close to the correct pronunciation as possible, but we would like to apologize to our readers who are Indian-language speakers for the factual incorrectness of this practice.

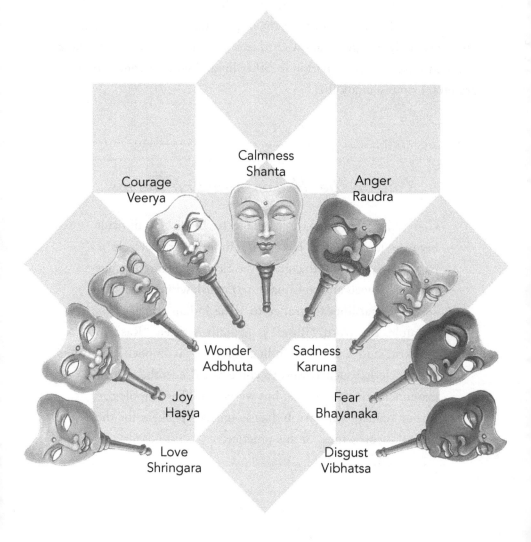

Calmness
Shanta

Courage
Veerya

Anger
Raudra

Wonder
Adbhuta

Sadness
Karuna

Joy
Hasya

Fear
Bhayanaka

Love
Shringara

Disgust
Vibhatsa

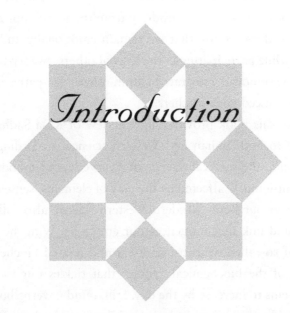

Introduction

Rasas are the essences of our emotions that exist in both body and mind. The Indian tradition recognizes nine Rasas as representing our most important and basic emotions: Love, Joy, Wonder, Courage, Calmness, Anger, Sadness, Fear, and Disgust. Some are desirable: the cream of life and the very purpose of creation. Others are unpleasant and most often not desirable.

Rasa Sadhana is the Yoga of the Nine Emotions, increasing understanding and exercising control over various flavors of happiness. For example, by temporarily promising ourselves not to be angry in thought, word, and deed, we may come to a better understanding of the Anger Rasa and master it to such extent that we become really free to express Anger or not. Similar vows may be adopted for a lifetime and can provide us with very special powers. Others may be hard to maintain even for one day, but will provide valuable insight and control just the same. Such "Rasa fasts" are of great help in learning to dissolve unpleasant emotions without suppressing them.

Every imaginable desire ultimately aims at some happy feeling that we expect to enjoy when fulfilling that desire. Rasa Sadhana allows us to pursue happiness more directly and durably. Rasa Yoga is especially useful to the householder who tries to live a spiritual life in modern society. It does not ask us to withdraw from the world, nor does it consume time. It does require that we remain emotionally and spiritually disciplined while participating in the lives of others, twenty-four hours a day. It can be smoothly integrated within other yoga paths and is easily taught by advanced yoga teachers.

Part 1 of this book provides an overview of Rasa Sadhana and its relationship to both Indian and Western science. According to Indian philosophy and the medical science of Ayurveda, our moods and emotions are continuously affected by the play of elements, senses, food, and vital energy in our body. Modern Western science also fully supports the body-mind link that influences our emotions. With the continuing discovery of so-called neurotransmitters and related biochemicals, the complexity of the biochemical "soup" that tickles our thoughts and emotions seems to increase by the day. Still, mind governs body and not vice versa, unless we allow it. Indian philosophy further offers a clear insight into the interactions between the Rasas and our mind, intellect, ego, and self.

An in-depth study of each of the nine Rasas is the main subject of Part 2 of this book. Each Rasa has basic expressions found in both ancient and modern times. They correspond to particular psychological and biochemical environments. Some sub-Rasas exist and each Rasa has clear relationships to other Rasas, allowing us to strengthen or weaken one Rasa through another. In addition to describing these attributes and relationships, Part 2 introduces practical as well as philosophical ways to gain control over each Rasa, specifically in the form of guidelines for the corresponding Rasa Sadhana or emotional fasting exercise.

Part 3 combines all this knowledge into practical advice on working with our emotions in daily life. Rasas of preference are defined depending on personal history, talent, and body type. The conditions for successfully exercising emotional control are established and each of the senses becomes a window through which emotions can be given new directions. As food strongly affects our biochemical receptivity to happy emotions, the basic rules for emotionally healthy cooking are given. Daily routines strengthen and balance physical and emotional well-being. In case of emotional emergencies, a number of clear steps may put us back on the road to happiness.

As the Rasas are strongly tied to our relationships with others and with society in general, Part 4 helps us to understand the emotional evolution of humankind. Modern science will bring us many new findings on the subject that may be valuable or not. Yoga and other spiritual sciences are of great help and likewise Rasa Sadhana is very useful for easier advancement along the many yogic paths, allowing for more fruitful meditation and deeper devotion. Traditionally, the Indian arts have provided society with the subtle treat of more refined feelings and modern artists have a similar role to play. Advertising has been stirring desire by playing on our emotions for decades. New "mood foods" and other mood-related products may further lead to the commercialization of happiness that disturbs our view of reality. Part 4 offers insights about these influences and how to make wholesome choices among them, as well as indicating how the knowledge of Rasas can be successfully applied in therapy, such that the therapist becomes a real teacher.

Sometimes feelings of anger, worry, sadness, or depression fall upon us, even though we dislike them. Sometimes we long for love, joy, courage, wonder, or peace, but seem unable to produce these enjoyable feelings. The ancient Indian knowledge and practical exercises described in this book can help anyone to become a master of his or her emotions.

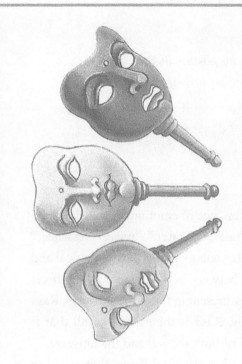

PART ONE

Rasa Sadhana

1

Nine Rasas

The most difficult posture in
yoga is the ever-changing posture of daily life.

The Sanskrit word Rasa means "the essence of emotion," as well as having more literal meanings such as "taste," "water," "juice," "essence," and ultimately "bliss." Rasa is a kind of energy that is partly physical and partly mental. It is an important link between body and mind that affects our thoughts and emotions. As energy present in the entire universe, Rasa affects us as gravity affects our body. Rasa is the essence of all that is inside and outside, the feeling nature of both the self and the universe.

The Indian tradition recognizes nine principal Rasas that relate to quite clearly defined moods or emotions:

THE NINE RASAS

Sanskrit Term	Principal Meaning	Further Meanings and Related Emotions
Shringara	Love	Beauty, Aesthetic Sentiment, Devotion
Hasya	Joy	Humor, Laughter, Sarcasm
Adbhuta	Wonder	Curiosity, Astonishment, Mystery

Sanskrit Term	Principal Meaning	Further Meanings and Related Emotions
Shanta	Calmness	Peace, Relaxation, Rest
Raudra	Anger	Violence, Irritation, Stress
Veerya	Courage	Heroism, Determination, Confidence
Karuna	Sadness	Compassion, Pity, Sympathy
Bhayanaka	Fear	Terror, Anxiety, Nervousness, Worry
Vibhatsa	Disgust	Depression, Dissatisfaction, Self-Pity

Rasa is the essential aspect of a set of emotions and moods that belong to the same "family." When a Rasa is present for some time, its energy affects the body and mind in such a way that one of the members of its family of emotions is manifested. The Adbhuta or Wonder Rasa, for example, can manifest as curiosity, astonishment, or mystery. Bhayanaka or Fear can manifest as terror, anxiety, nervousness, or worry.

In the case of three of the Rasas, two meanings are so significant that they are often used almost interchangeably: Shringara as Love and Beauty; Hasya as Joy and Humor; and Karuna as Sadness and Compassion. However, in each case, one of the meanings is more inclusive: Joy can exist without Humor, while Humor cannot exist without Joy; Compassion always holds an element of Sadness (would not the saint that feels Compassion prefer not to have to feel it, in an ideal world?), while Sadness can exist without an element of Compassion; Love can exist without any element of Beauty (one can love a both physically and mentally truly ugly and disgusting person), while to admire the Beauty of somebody or something always produces a feeling of Love toward it. So Love, Sadness, and Joy are the true Rasas or essences.

While the Rasas themselves are clearly defined energies, the resulting emotions (Bhavas) manifest in many varieties and their understanding is affected by personal and cultural backgrounds. For example, the Anger Rasa produces Bhavas such as irritation, anger, and fury. In this book, we pay little attention to the difference between Rasa and Bhava, because both phenomena basically occur together. However, there is a more extensive discussion of the differences between Rasa and Bhava in chapter 23 on art.

Desirable and Less Desirable Rasas

Whether a Rasa is desirable or not depends on the situation. One can say that some Rasas are agreeable (Love, Joy, Courage, Calmness, Wonder) and others are not (Anger, Fear, Sadness, Disgust). However, even Anger can be agreeable if one really feels it is justified and Joy may not always be appropriate, such as at a funeral. Nevertheless, in general terms, Anger, Fear, Sadness, and Disgust are neither desirable nor agreeable, while the other Rasas are agreeable and desirable.

Sometimes we have no idea why a particular Rasa catches us and sometimes its origin is very clear. Things that happen around us can trigger a Rasa, as well as our inner thoughts and unconscious associations. Rasas are strongly connected with our relationships; the more important those relationships are, the stronger our emotions may become. We can only really hate somebody we love. Rasas may overpower our entire personality, sweeping away all reason in just a second. Often we desire to leave a particular mood but seem powerless to direct our emotional state.

In Indian art, a painting or a play is complete when all Rasas are present in proper proportion. The same goes for life itself. Without Rasas, life is *ni-rasa* ("no-Rasa"), empty of the juice or moisture that gives taste to life, leaving it barren, dry, dull, boring, and dead. The Rasas create variety in the theater of life. If there is no Disgust, then there can be no Beauty. If there is no Joy, then Sadness cannot be recognized. As the purpose of Indian art is to create Rasa in the spectators, Indian artists have been very important in the development of the science of Rasas, as further explored in chapter 23.

Rasa Sadhana

We can be slaves of our Rasas or not. All emotions make sense sometimes, but not at all times. Agreeable Rasas usually create positive desires that elevate our consciousness and lead to agreeable Rasas in turn. Less agreeable Rasas often create negative desires that degrade our consciousness and lead to less agreeable Rasas.

All desires for ownership, security, enjoyment, recognition, love, knowledge, enlightenment, and so on are desires for the happiness that we hope to feel by fulfilling them. For example, when somebody buys a big car to impress his or her neighbors, the objective is not the impressing itself but the feeling that it may produce. Whatever form the desire takes, feeling happy is all that we ever really desire. Should happiness then not be pursued more directly and durably? That is the essential objective of Rasa Sadhana, which literally means "emotional discipline."

Rasas are the essential drive of our existence, yet Rasas are the subject about which we are the most ignorant and over which most of us seem to have the least control. Rasa Sadhana offers increased control over the Rasas through:

❖ Understanding the relationships between different Rasas, and between Rasas and the body and various aspects of life.
❖ Exercises that teach Rasa control and increase real understanding of each Rasa, through a kind of emotional fasting.

Rasa Sadhana is "Rasa fasting" in the sense that it includes fasting from or on specific emotions. For example, we first promise ourselves that for a day or a week or longer we will not get involved with one of the less desirable Rasas, such as Anger, Fear, Sadness, or Disgust. When the emotion surfaces it will not be suppressed, but properly analyzed; that alone will render it largely powerless. With the aid of some specific techniques that often involve the body, the energy of the Rasa can be more fully dissolved. The promise made in the Sadhana will provide us with the willpower to do so in any case, because to fail means to hurt the ego and when the ego gets involved the Rasa stands no chance. Through such regular exercise, we rapidly learn that we really can master these emotions quite effortlessly.

When the less desirable Rasas have thus been brought under control, we can start fasting on the desirable Rasas, such as Calmness, Love, Joy, Wonder, and Courage. For a particular length of time set by the practitioner, willpower is used to stay in the chosen Rasa, regardless of what happens. Each Rasa is always present in every situation, so we can learn to extract it from whatever happens. Through such Rasa Sadhana, anybody can become a true Rasa master. While it may seem that we have little impact on the things that happen to us, we are always fully in charge of our emotional reactions to them. We have every right to be happy or unhappy and can develop the power to exercise that right. Just as nobody can stop us from feeling unhappy unless we allow it, nobody can stop us from having happy feelings if we have properly exercised our capacity for them.

Rasa Sadhana also provides the serious practitioner with special powers called *siddhis*. Their nature and importance are discussed in relation to each Rasa in Part 2.

Rasa Sadhana is a kind of yoga that is practiced in life itself rather than by withdrawal from life. It especially offers spiritual exercise to the householder who has not withdrawn from life but lives it and wants to live it. Although the practice of Rasa Sadhana is very ancient, it has been so fully integrated within other yoga branches that it has become somewhat invisible. It originated in the time before Hindu yogis started organizing themselves into more institutionalized *akaras* (schools) and *ashrams* (communities). This major change in Hinduism happened as a reaction to the growing popularity of the Buddhist monasteries in the fourth and third centuries BCE. Before that time, spiritual teaching happened in the *gurukula,* the family home of the teacher. These teachers were usually married and had children, so the teaching that took place connected directly to normal life.

Even though complete withdrawal from this world may be the grand finale of the game of life *(leela)* and even though temporary withdrawal is an essential tool for spiritual growth, God did not create this world so that everybody would run away from it immediately. Life must be enjoyed and experienced to realize its true purpose. Many people in India feel that sadhana inside the world is more truthful than sadhana performed when removed from the world. To be detached from something that is not present seems easier than to be detached in the face of full temptation. In fact, the truthfulness of sadhana depends solely on the person who is performing it, whether in the world or outside of it. Withdrawing to a cave while still thinking of the wide world around it makes no sense and neither does living in the world while dreaming of a cave.

A real saint has mastered all Rasas, even if Calmness is the preferred Rasa. He or she is not only ever peaceful, but also full of Love and Joy, always humbly conscious of the divine Wonder that is ever around and courageous in his or her disciplines. A saint does not react in Anger, Fear, or Disgust, although Compassion (Karuna) can be an attribute (see chapter 11). He or she may not have obtained this control over the Rasas through Rasa Sadhana, but naturally through any of the many other spiritual paths.

If saints become fathers and mothers after achieving very deep states of meditation, they might be able to keep their inner peace within close reach. However, without such depth of experience, even strongly spiritual householders and parents can hardly ever maintain the Calmness Rasa for a prolonged period. Their responsibilities simply do not allow it. They can experience moments of deep peace every day if they want, but daily life will not allow them to fully hold on to it.

Rasa Sadhana offers an alternative spiritual path, which includes the Calmness Rasa, but also teaches us to find happiness and spiritual growth in the other Rasas. It teaches us to master all Rasas so that we may at least choose the Rasa that we desire, usually one of the generally agreeable Rasas. The trio of Love, Wonder, and Joy can be enjoyed with near and dear ones, as well as in relation to the universe and the Divine. The fearlessness and focus offered by the Courage Rasa help to support us and foster our personal discipline. Compassion may lead to selfless service and it is always possible to find some time and the right frame of mind for some deep Calmness. Through Rasa Sadhana, householders may more easily accept the limitations that are their *karma* (destiny) and *dharma* (duty). When their children become self-sufficient, they may still leave the world and chose the path of the renunciate, as do so many older people in India. There, it is quite common for an elderly person to leave his or her family, home, and occupation to search for a more spiritual life by undertaking a long pilgrimage or living in an ashram.

Rasa Sadhana is a particularly interesting spiritual discipline for people living in modern society. It does not require stepping outside of social life, nor does it require any extra time investment. Not being angry, sad, disgusted, or worried requires no extra time, so this kind of yoga is very useful to the householder, who may have only an hour a day or so to practice meditation. If we can remain free from disturbing emotions during the day, then the meditation that we are able to do will be much more fruitful.

Rasa Sadhana combines the knowledge of various ancient Indian sciences. It is primarily tantric in origin, Tantra being a holistic approach to the study of the universal from the point of view of the individual and highly specialized in the art of reprogramming ourselves. Rasa Sadhana also draws heavily on Ayurveda, the science of life that imparts practical as well as medical knowledge. It is based also on yogic philosophy and the wisdom of the original Vedas, as well as on somewhat less ancient Hindu scriptures.

2

Rasas in the Body

*Emotions are experienced as a play of elements
and energies in the body.*

Rasas are neither purely physical nor purely mental. In Tantra, each body cell has a "mind" of its own. Body and mind really are one.

Bad body chemistry creates disagreeable Rasas and a healthy body offers the basis for more happy Rasas. If a particular Rasa is fed with thoughts and ideas that support it, a persistent biochemical environment in the body is created or strengthened. That body chemistry will cause the Rasa to remain for a longer period. Even if the person is temporarily distracted from that Rasa, the moment the distraction ends, the Rasa will come back. This is true for both agreeable and disagreeable Rasas.

When a disagreeable Rasa catches us for a long period, the biochemical environment created in our body is difficult to get rid of and may lead to disease. Maintaining an agreeable Rasa over a long period will stabilize our body, keeping it healthy and curing disease.

According to the science of Ayurveda, Rasas relate to: the five elements; the three *doshas* (humors or temperaments); the three *gunas* (energy qualities of nature); the seven *dhatus* (constituents of the human body); the five senses; food; *prana* (the vital life force), and the seven *chakras* (energy centers).

Rasas and Elements

According to Hindu philosophy, the phenomenal world is a play of five elements: earth, water, fire, air, and akasha (ether or space). They are the materialized form of the universal energy that vibrates at ever-denser levels.

Without food, the fruit of the earth element, we can only survive for weeks. Without water, our lifespan becomes a matter of days. Without heat or the element of fire, our body can only sustain itself for a few hours, and without air, normal people die within minutes. Without space, not even seconds are available. Therefore, without earth, water, fire, air, and space, life is impossible.

Although water is the primary element of Rasa, fire and air are also involved in the play of the Rasas in the body. Certain Rasas are more closely affiliated with particular elements, as shown:

DOMINANT ELEMENTS OF THE RASAS

Water	Fire	Air
Love	Joy	Calmness
Courage	Wonder	Fear
Sadness	Anger	
Disgust		

However, just as the elements never appear in a pure form, the Rasas also do not depend solely on one element. Rasas dominated by the air or fire elements still have water, because water is the primary element of all Rasas. The elements represent an evolution from subtle to gross, with water containing air and fire, and fire also containing air. These three elements are thus present in every Rasa, in varying proportions.

Rasas and Doshas

In our body, the five elements assume the form of three doshas (humors): *kapha* (mucus), *pitta* (bile), and *vata* (wind). It is through the understanding of the doshas that the science of Ayurveda studies the play of the elements in the body. Dosha literally means "fault" so the focus is on the factors that cause imbalance and disease, whether physical or mental.

Each dosha combines two elements: kapha contains water and earth; pitta contains fire and water; vata contains air and akasha. Our physical and emotional health depends on the proper balance of the three doshas in the body. When they are in balance, each dosha produces a subtle energy essence; when they are disturbed, they create the following disagreeable Rasas:

DISTURBED DOSHAS AND RASAS

Kapha (Mucus)	Pitta (Bile)	Vata (Wind)
Sadness	Anger	Fear
Disgust		

Kapha is the most important dosha for the production of harmonious feelings. It is primarily produced in the stomach, from where it provides nutritional fluids throughout the body. When kapha is in balance, it produces *ojas* (primary vigor), which is its essence. Disturbed kapha causes Sadness and Disgust.

Pitta is a very thin fluid, hot in nature, like bile. If it is disturbed, then Anger will only need a spark to explode. If pitta is in balance, it makes us smart and radiant through its essence, which is called *tejas* (inner radiance).

Vata is generally regarded as the most important of the three doshas. Pitta and kapha need the air of vata to move them to their required places throughout the body. Disturbed vata, often caused by constipation, may thus lead not only to Fear, but also to Anger, Sadness, and Disgust. When vata is in perfect balance, it is converted to its essence, which is prana, and produces Calmness.

Prana, tejas, and ojas—the subtle essences of vata, pitta, and kapha, respectively—exist beyond the physical level. There is a strong relationship between these subtle essences of the doshas and the development of the higher aspects of the Rasas, such as universal love, true compassion, absolute fearlessness, and innocent joy. Prana, tejas, and ojas can only durably emerge if all three doshas are properly balanced.

Rasas and Gunas

The gunas are the three main qualities that are present at the core of every phenomenon. Together with the five elements, the three gunas constitute the eight-fold nature of manifested reality. These all-pervading forces or qualities of energy are:

❖ Sattva: light; stands for clarity, understanding, and healing
❖ Rajas: movement; stands for inspiration, activity, and pain
❖ Tamas: inertia; stands for doubt, darkness, and attachment

Each Rasa is dominated by one guna:

DOMINANT GUNAS OF THE RASAS

Sattva	Rajas	Tamas
Calmness	Love	Disgust
	Joy	Fear
	Wonder	
	Courage	
	Sadness	
	Anger	

Fear usually makes a person dull, inactive, frozen, or tamasic, but has a more rajasic expression in hysteria. Love is by nature rajasic, but can have a more sattvic nature in art or spiritual devotion. Joy as Humor is rajasic by nature, but may become more sattvic if it is very innocent or more tamasic if it is sarcastic. These subtle variations in each Rasa will become clearer in Part 2.

Food, Senses, and Rasas

Food and the senses are the primary channels through which the environment affects the Rasas via the intermediary of the physical body.

The effect of foods on the Rasas depends on three actions: taste (rasa), power during digestion *(virya)*, and post-digestive action *(vipaka)*. While taste causes the most immediate effect, the effects during and after digestion are a lot more durable. Foods thus directly affect the doshas that promote various Rasas, as explained above.

On an energy level, the three gunas provide us with great insight on how to control the Rasas through food and the senses:

❖ Tamasic Rasas can be affected by the input of rajas through the senses or through food. For example, Fear may be replaced more easily by Courage through the ingestion of pungent foods, which are rajasic in nature.

❖ Rajasic Rasas can be affected by the input of sattva, such as Anger being more rapidly calmed down by meditative music.

❖ Sattvic Rasas can be affected by the input of both rajas and tamas: a calm mood may easily be disturbed by the intake of too much sugar (rajas) and fat (tamas) in a chocolate bar.

In chapter 3, we will further explore the relationships between Rasas, foods, and senses.

Rasas, Prana, and Breath

Prana is the vital air that creates all action in both the body and the mind. While it enters the body with the air that we breathe, prana is not simply oxygen or negative ions, but the life force that is contained by air.

The Rasas are produced in the body and mind by the interaction of prana with the doshas, that is, the activation of the elements through the life force. Slow breathing (especially stopping the breath for some time) stops this process; it stops the mind and will change the Rasa if maintained for a sufficiently long period.

Breath also affects the Rasas by way of the two energy channels known as *nadis*. Each of the two hemispheres of the brain is activated by the nadi associated with it. At any given time one of our two nostrils may be dominant in our breathing, which stimulates its respective nadi, and thus its related side of the brain. The Ida Nadi—which is lunar and emotional in nature—relates to the right side of the brain and is stimulated by left nostril breathing. The Pingala Nadi—which is solar and rational in nature—relates to the left side of the brain and right nostril breathing. Swar Yoga* (a yoga based on the science of breath) and *pranayama* (conscious breath control) techniques thus offer powerful tools to control body chemistry and the Rasas.

Rasas and Chakras

Chakras are subtle energy centers that are located along the spine. Each chakra corresponds to a particular element, as well as to a basic desire, certain behavioral characteristics, and a stage of spiritual development. The study of the chakras is the main subject of Kundalini Yoga, which has the objective of waking the *kundalini* ("serpent-power") energy that lies dormant in the first chakra at the base of the spine. Special techniques are used to move this energy upward to pierce each of the chakras in turn, until in the seventh chakra enlightenment is reached. The table on the following page shows the location of each chakra as well as its related element and desire.

A person who resides primarily in one or the other of the chakras is mostly dominated by the basic desire that relates to that chakra. All people, except very small children, are active within the first three chakras. Some also move into the higher chakras. Much more information about chakras and Kundalini Yoga can be found in Harish Johari's book on chakras.[†]

---

*For more information on the nadis and Swar Yoga, see: Harish Johari, *Breath, Mind, and Consciousness* (Rochester, Vt.: Destiny Books, 1989).
†Harish Johari, *Chakras* (Rochester, Vt.: Destiny Books, 2000).

THE SEVEN CHAKRAS

Chakra	Location	Element	Basic Desire
First Chakra (Muladhara Chakra)	Pelvic plexus	Earth	Security
Second Chakra (Svadhishthana Chakra)	Hypogastric plexus	Water	Enjoyment
Third Chakra (Manipura Chakra)	Solar plexus	Fire	Status
Fourth Chakra (Anahata Chakra)	Cardiac plexus	Air	Balance
Fifth Chakra (Vishuddha Chakra)	Carotid plexus	Akasha (Ether)	Knowledge
Sixth Chakra (Ajna Chakra)	Pineal plexus	Mahatattva (supreme or great element in which all other elements are present in essence)	Enlightenment
Seventh Chakra (Sahasrara Chakra)	Cerebral plexus	Beyond Elements	Beyond Desires

As explained earlier, Rasas are dominated by the water element, so they all primarily relate to the second chakra. There is no one-to-one correspondence between the chakras and particular Rasas. However, the level of spiritual development associated with a person's dominating chakra determines the quality of the expression of each Rasa. The Anger of a person dominated by the first chakra will be mostly caused by fears and insecurities, while that of a third chakra person will mostly relate to pride and concerns about status. The Love of a second chakra person may be rather sensuous, while that of a fourth chakra person will be related to desires for family union, and that of a sixth chakra person more universal. Further discussion about these variations will be found in Part 2.

3

Body Emotions in Western Science

*In the study of body-mind relationships, modern science
is centuries behind but rapidly gaining speed.*

It is often hard to accept that thoughts, moods, and emotions have any-thing to do with our body, because we tend to regard them as sincere and unique. Any relation made between them and the body, the environ-ment, or our food is easily regarded as a rather horrific attack on our personality. Even though Western society likes to regard body and mind as being strictly separated, some exceptions have been acknowledged for a long time, such as psychosomatic diseases (caused by psychological problems) and psychoactive drugs. Fortunately, during the past couple of decades, Western science has produced more proof of a deep relation-ship between body and mind. This research has led to the development of modern tranquilizers and antidepressants such as Prozac.

Modern Western knowledge primarily has value in demonstrating the connection between body and mind, but offers us very little in terms of practical advice about how to control the mind. Since Western science seems so very convincing to modern minds, it can help us to once and for all accept that our thoughts and emotions are heavily colored by our body chemistry. But the approaches of Yoga, Tantra, and Ayurveda offer much more practical insight and advice about how to really work with our mind through our body.

The Functioning of the Brain

Some of the major centers of the brain take part in regulating our emotions. The forebrain—the largest part of the brain—is primarily made up of the cerebrum, which is divided into two hemispheres. The surface of each hemisphere is made up of gray matter known as the cerebral cortex. The cortex controls perception, memory, and all higher cognitive functions, including the ability to concentrate, reason, and think in abstract form. Nerve pulses from the right part of the body mostly end up in the left side of the cerebrum and vice versa. The left hemisphere mostly handles rational thought while the right hemisphere takes care of emotional and intuitive thought.

The forebrain also includes several other major centers that are involved with our emotions, such as the thalamus, the hypothalamus, and the limbic system. The thalamus functions to relay sensory information to the cerebral cortex and the hypothalamus regulates visceral functions, such as temperature, reproductive functions, eating, sleeping, and the display of emotion. The limbic system—which includes the amygdala and hippocampus—is also known as the "emotional brain," as it is important in the formation of memories and in controlling emotions, decisions, motivation, and learning.

The main task of nerve cells is to transfer messages as electric pulses to other nerve cells in our brain and body, using channels called dendrites and neurites. These are extremely thin, thread-like "branches" that connect every nerve cell to other nerve cells. Dendrites are used for receiving signals and neurites for sending them.

Information Molecules

The neurites and dendrites of nerve cells do not directly connect to each other. Between them there are spaces known as synapses, which are filled with the cerebrospinal fluid in which all brain tissue is embedded. The electric pulse that is sent from one nerve cell to another does not simply flow through this fluid. The transfer of the information in the electric pulse happens with the help of molecules in the cerebrospinal fluid called neurotransmitters. These neurotransmitters absorb and pass on the information. Therefore, all that we think or feel reflects a countless series of electrical and biochemical signals.

Neurotransmitters are also essential in the transfer of information from nerve cells to other body cells and vice versa. To read the information contained in these neurotransmitters, all body cells have "receptor molecules," attached like long antenna to the outside of their cellular bodies. Neurotransmitters, receptor molecules, and substances that affect them are today grouped as "information molecules."

SOME OF THE
BEST-KNOWN INFORMATION MOLECULES

Information Molecules	Influence on	Related to
Acetylcholine	concentration	nicotine
Adrenalin	fight-or-flight response, nervousness	meat
Cortical Releasing Factor	depression and stress	suicide
Cholycystokinin	satisfaction	tryptophane
Dopamine	fear, alertness	cocaine, clozapine
Endorphin	joy, love, sadness, pain	opium, heroin, sugar
Phenylethylamine	joy, love, depression, paranoia	chocolate, falling in love
GABA	nervousness	valium
Melatonin	nervousness, sleep	melatonin drug
Noradrenalin	aggression, fear, depression, cheerfulness	amphetamine, cocaine, caffeine
Oxytocin	love and satisfaction	orgasm

Information Molecules	Influence on	Related to
Progesterone	inner peace and love	pregnancy
Serotonin	inner peace, depression, nervousness	Prozac, Ecstasy, LSD

The first neurotransmitters were discovered in the 1950s: acetylcholine, noradrenalin, dopamine, and serotonin. In the 60s followed the amino acids of the GABA-type and in the 70s the peptides. Later it also became clear that hormones act as neurotransmitters and affect neurotransmitters.

Drugs, Senses, and Food

All known drugs relate to natural and often similar information molecules in our body. The body's own endorphins are very similar to morphine, the active compound of heroin. THC in cannabis, or marijuana, relates to the anandamides in our body, even though that is certainly not the only type of neurotransmitter involved. Serotonin in our body relates to Prozac and Ecstasy.

Information molecules are directly affected by sensory input and in their turn these molecules also affect sensory perception. We not only hear, see, taste, touch, and smell with our ears, eyes, tongue, skin, and nose, but also with our entire body, through the information molecules. Likewise, sensory input not only affects our brain, but our entire body and hence our emotions as well.

Modern science also teaches that foods affect our information molecules and thus our emotional state. The taste of foods immediately affects our levels of various neurotransmitters. Our intestines are lined with receptors for neurotransmitters, so the effects during digestion of the neurotransmitters in foods are immediate and only partly reduced by digestion. After digestion, foods clearly affect blood chemistry; our brains are completely penetrated by blood vessels that determine the composition of the cerebrospinal fluid, which is replaced several times a day. Obviously not all blood components are transferred to the cerebrospinal fluid, but many neurotransmitters are.

Drugs that people use compete with the body's own "drugs" or information molecules. If drugs are taken in large amounts, the specific receptors for those information molecules are overwhelmed, which causes their number and activity to decrease. When the direct effect of the drug is gone, our ability to get the same feelings through our own information molecules or natural body drugs is reduced. This attack on our natural ability to feel good may have short or prolonged effects, depending on the strength and type of drug used.

The typical definition for "drugs" is "substances that alter the mental state." The addictive effect is also supposed to distinguish drugs from other substances and processes that affect our mind. In fact, all external influences on the body have drug-like effects, from music to the smell of roses or a cup of coffee. The example of drugs teaches us to be careful when using any external factor, such as music, special herbs, foods, and so on in order to affect our emotions. If we commonly use external factors to make ourselves "happy," our natural ability to feel good will be reduced. This does not mean that external factors cannot be used, but that moderation and diversity make a lot of sense. In any case, external factors cannot be completely avoided, but we can be careful in dealing with their quality and quantity.

Emotional Patterns

One of the most fantastic findings of science is that we are continuously creating new connections between nerve cells, by creating new neurites and dendrites. Our thinking thus continuously creates new neural patterns, pathways of communication between parts of the brain and also of the body. They largely determine our reaction to what happens to us. The more we use a particular pattern, the broader the pathway becomes. Some backstreet alleys of our brain may thus develop into real highways and vice versa. Thus, reprogramming our brain has never been science fiction—it happens all the time.

Every neural pattern reflects as a biochemical pattern in our body. Such a pattern consists of particular mixtures of information molecules spread throughout specific parts of the body. In people with strong emotional blocks, exceptional biochemical patterns are found, primarily among the receptors on body cells. These receptors truly represent the emotional memory of the body, another major factor determining our reactions to life.

Rasa Sadhana offers a clear method to effectively change these emotional, neural, and biochemical reaction patterns.

4

Indian Philosophy and Rasas

Let not the power of the body become an excuse
for not staying on top of it.

Even though body chemistry is a very useful tool in controlling the Rasas, the mental approach is far more important. Mind governs body and not vice versa, unless we allow it. Understanding the body-mind relationship should not be used as a self-fulfilling prophecy. For example, if your body has become tamasic (lazy) because of illness, junk food, or excessive sensory indulgences, it is not a given that you have to feel bad. Feeling good or bad always remains a personal choice.

According to Hindu philosophy, individual consciousness is a partial expression of cosmic consciousness. Cosmic consciousness and individual consciousness are one; only subjectivity separates them. Consciousness is the ultimate reality out of which both the mental and the material proceed.

When consciousness manifests as an organism, it needs tools to control and work with the physical body. Hindu philosophy uses a model of the human organism that consists of five such tools regarded as sheaths *(koshas)*. This same model is also used in Ayurvedic psychology, where it serves in therapeutic analysis. The koshas form one of the basic concepts of Hindu philosophy—which regards the individual and the cosmos as one—so it would be incorrect to regard them only as psychological terms.

Sheath of Self or Bliss *(Anandamaya Kosha)*

All other sheaths fold like onion layers around the central point, which contains the Self *(chitta)*. The Self dwells in our spiritual heart, which is "located" to the right of our physical heart. The Self is usually not consciously experienced, although it is always present and can be experienced at any moment. The Self is the true "I" that witnesses whatever happens. The Self is also bliss: Nothing is disturbing to the Self, because nothing is real to the Self. The Self is the Truth and that Truth is never changing. The Self is the screen upon which the movie of life is played and which remains white after the movie is over. The Self is our divine spark of consciousness, our "little" god inside.

The Hindu God Shiva represents the divine lover (consciousness and the Self) while his spouse Shakti is the beloved (energy, the body, and the phenomenal world). Their relationship is beautifully expressed in the following conversation:

> Shakti creates a world of her own and invites Shiva inside. "Hey, I have created a world, will you come?" Shiva says, "Sure, but I cannot live in it, because it is ever changing and I am never changing, so what should I do?" She replies, "If you get into everything as the center of everything, then the center never changes, only everything around it changes. You are always surrounded by eternal bliss; you remain in your bliss. Around you, I will put a network of my powers that will intermediate between you and the outside world. That way you will not have to do anything. You can remain never changing and I can remain ever changing and we can have fun." Shiva agrees, and the game of life starts.

Sheath of Ego and Intellect *(Vijnanamaya Kosha)*

This sheath is the sheath of knowledge beyond sense perception, which combines the ego and the intellect and travels with the Self from one body to the next.

Ego is the tool of consciousness that links all events in life together. Ego is the illusion that "I exist as a separate individual being." Ego is the one that assumes responsibility for the body and identifies with it. Ego also identifies with the character or personality created out of past and future actions. Ego also manages relationships with the world outside, through attachment and detachment.

The intellect represents our memory and our ability to draw conclusions from past experiences. It stores whatever we have experienced in this life or in past lives. The intellect gets a part of the genetic information from seven generations of the father's side and from seven generations of the mother's side. The intellect advises the ego.

Sheath of Mind *(Manomaya Kosha)*

Mind is the tool of consciousness that enables us to perceive the world and process the incoming information. The world exists for us only because of our five senses. The mind uses the brain as one of its main tools, but it also pervades everything, every body cell. It has no specific seat. This "mind" of the body cells is scientific fact today. The cells' main tools of "thought" are the "information molecules" mentioned earlier: neurotransmitters, the substances that affect neurotransmitters, and the receptor molecules attached to cells (see chapter 3). The functions of the body thus extend far beyond that of "carrying our thinking brain."

The mind is the greatest obstacle in the way of rational thinking. Similarly, if one tries to sit and remain silent inside, then the first obstacle is the mind, which jumps from one subject to another by association.

Sheath of Vital Air *(Pranamaya Kosha)*

The sheath of vital air supplies energy as prana to the whole system and keeps it alive. The breath provides the pranic force to the organism; however, prana refers not only to the flow of oxygen, but also to the life force that is contained by it. This energy enters each pore and every cell. The breath is the physical counterpart of the mind. All sensory and motor functions of the body are performed with the help of the breath. This pranic force, working as the air element, creates movement, pulsation, vibration, and life.

Sheath of Matter *(Annamaya Kosha)*

The sheath of matter that represents our cellular body contains all other sheaths. It is created from the elements in food *(anna)*. The main parts of the body that connect to the other koshas are the brain, the spine, the nerves and other subtle channels (nadis), the five sense organs (eyes, ears, nose, tongue, skin), and the five work organs (anus, genitals, legs, hands, vocal chords).

Rasas, Indian Philosophy, and Psychology

Our body is a kingdom, with the ego as the king, intellect as the prime minister, mind as the government administration, and the Self as God. Most of the time, the country is governed by the administration or mind. Whenever something unusual needs to be decided, the king (ego) is advised by the prime minister (intellect) and then makes a decision. Unfortunately, the king is often confused by the amount of information brought to him by the administration (mind) and by attachment to and identification with the kingdom (body). As a result, the king (ego) often does not properly listen to the wise prime minister (intellect). God (the Self) remains unaffected by whatever happens.

By the interaction of prana with the doshas in the body, the Rasas are experienced in the mind. At that point, ego has to decide if it accepts the Rasa that is experienced. If the ego, after consulting the intellect, does not support a Rasa, then it will be changed by an act of willpower. If the ego supports a Rasa, then even the intellect can do nothing and may be forced by the ego to support the Rasa. Rasas are primarily a game of body and mind, but ego is still the key to controlling them. If a Rasa remains for a long period, it is because both the ego and the body support it.

All Rasas (except Calmness) relate primarily to body and mind, while in some Rasas the ego and intellect also play a major role:

RASAS AND KOSHAS

Rasa	Body and Mind	Ego	Intellect
Love	x	x	x
Joy	x		
Wonder	x		
Calmness			
Anger	x	x	x
Courage	x	x	x
Sadness	x	x	x
Fear	x	x	x
Disgust	x		

The above table is relevant only to the Rasas in their pure form. When, for example, a scientist suddenly understands some aspect of his study, it produces a "Eureka!" feeling that belongs to the Wonder Rasa, but is not pure Wonder because of the involvement of the intellect. Likewise, when a strong feeling of Joy comes, its force and purity will decrease the moment one becomes conscious of thinking "I am feeling *great*," even though the ego involvement will not make the Rasa disappear entirely. The purest Calmness can only be experienced when neither mind, nor ego, nor intellect is active, which only happens to people that can experience *samadhi*, the highest state of meditation. Of course, other people can experience the Calmness Rasa as well, but in a less pure form.

Throughout everything that happens, the Self (chitta) is the witnessing consciousness. It is aware of what happens, but it does not enter the play of emotions. Bliss is the primordial feeling or true Rasa of which all others are but manifestations. It always exists at the heart of one's being, where all Rasas merge into one. The Rasas dwell within the bliss that is chitta, but without association to particular emotions or moods (Bhavas), as essences that remain as pure as the chitta itself, mixed together in full harmony.

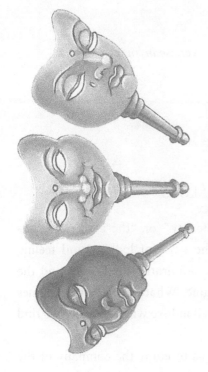

PART TWO

The Nine Rasas

5

Shringara: Love

To love one is an enchanting exercise in loving all.

The Basis of Love

Shringara means both "Love" and "Beauty" or "the aesthetic sentiment." A romantic atmosphere and the sense of looking and feeling
good enhance Love and harmony. The admiration of Beauty and the
Love for harmony are essentially the same. Whatever we love becomes
beautiful in our eyes and we naturally fall in love with whatever we find
beautiful, visually or otherwise.

Narrowly speaking, Shringara means to enjoy the company of the
opposite sex, in a very lovely and romantic manner. India's spiritual
epics are filled with love stories, with interludes such as when Krishna
and Radha are sitting together in a swing or when Rama puts flowers
in Sita's hair while they are in exile in the forest. Love and Beauty are
favorite subjects of stories, art, songs, literature, and poetry, as well as
common talk in every culture.

In a broader sense, Shringara is the mood in which we concentrate
on creating a lovely atmosphere, on family and friends, on good manners and romance, on art, culture, and decoration, on dressing attrac-

tively and behaving nicely, on Beauty and enjoyment. In Shringara the word "Rasa" most literally means "good taste." A master of Shringara is a master of the aesthetic sense, able to bring out the Beauty and harmony that is present in everything.

Various cultures have different understandings about what represents "good taste." For example, Indian women like to hear men say that they "walk like an elephant," because to Indian people elephants walk very elegantly. Indian men will be well advised not to say the same thing to Western women, however, because they might be quite offended. To them, elephants mostly have big behinds, which are not very popular in the West. The beautifully white and blissfully scented jasmine flowers that Indian lovers like to wear in their hair might, on the contrary, find approval anywhere.

Shringara is the Rasa Raj, the king of all Rasas, the super-Rasa. To some schools of Indian art it is the only Rasa. The Love Rasa stands closest to the bliss of the Self. Everybody experiences Shringara at least once in a lifetime. When we do not have the inner peace and bliss of a saint, what can we do without Love and Beauty? To concentrate on Love and Beauty means to worship the divinity of creation. Creation only happened for the enjoyment of Love, when Shiva and Shakti, the male and female energies, who were one, decided to play a game of hide and seek. Shringara thus can be understood as the very purpose of the universe.

Shringara is essential for physical, emotional, and spiritual health and growth, and in living a happy life. Love is the most extreme happiness that two people can create together, living as a god and goddess in a universe of their own. When two people harmonize their egos, the ego of each one becomes less important and the resulting shared ego of the couple may better balance male and female energies, attachments, and identifications. Surrender and serving each other are the keys to any good marriage or any other kind of stable love relationship. In this way the relationship becomes a rehearsal of surrender to the universe and the Divine; it is directly through such a close partnership of Love that this surrender may happen in its most exalted manner. Our universal Love may also be expressed in relationships with family, friends, and basically every person, animal, plant, or atom that we meet in life.

Mind is the dominant kosha (sheath) in Shringara, because it is our basic tool for experiencing both physical and mental enjoyment. The ego is also involved through the process of identification with the object of Shringara. The intellect may support it, for example by recalling sweet memories of earlier times spent with a loved one or by explaining the hidden meanings behind an object of art.

Artists play a very important role in stimulating the mood of Shringara. One might say that traditional artists are masters of Shringara. There is Beauty in everything, even in misery or ugliness. That Beauty can be appreciated through paintings, sculptures, drama, movies, the spectacle of natural beauty, and so on. As the spectator is not personally involved, even the most horrific or sad experience—when artfully expressed by an actor, musician, or artist—can create a feeling of enjoyment. More about the role of art can be read in chapter 23.

Shringara can be experienced on the physical, mental, and spiritual levels or on various combinations of these. Although Shringara can be experienced at all levels, it has a particular relationship with the second chakra. When it is experienced there, it is mostly physical and mental. When Shringara is experienced on the level of the fourth chakra, it may become very spiritual. Shringara can also be found in a more intellectual form, going into the world of meanings behind the aesthetic experience, which brings it to the fifth chakra level.

While everyone has the ability to live in Beauty and Love without much effort, most people seem to suffer from a lack of both. Partially this is due to the increased popularity of the Rasas that are "enemies" of Love, particularly Sadness, Anger, Fear, and Disgust (see the related chapters). It is also due to a real lack of understanding and appreciation of Shringara in modern culture. This is true in art and drama as well as in life.

Romantic feelings are no longer regarded as "cool," especially in Western society, and their cultural expression is mainly limited to movies for children and old ladies. The beneficial effects of art, decoration, music, and natural beauty on people's feelings are grossly underestimated. On the other hand, bodily beauty is totally overrated, with, for example, people choosing plastic surgery simply because their looks are not perfect. Moderation of sensual enjoyment is regarded as puritanical and as a result relationships suffer from exhaustion, excessive expectations, and boredom.

Sub-Rasas of Love

Many sub-Rasas of Shringara are recognized in which the Love is not between a man and a woman. The best-known and most revered sub-Rasa of Shringara in Indian society is the selfless and pure Love of a mother for her child. That parental Love is called the Vatsalya Rasa and can also be experienced when it is felt that the Divine requires nurturing worship. This usually finds expression in activities such as decorating a temple or cleaning and dressing up a statue of the deity.

The mood of Shringara has two aspects: The feeling of Love in union (Sambhoga Shringara) and in separation (Vipralambha Shringara). The problem with enjoying Love, as with every enjoyment, is that it has a tendency to become addictive. When the object of Love is not present, Love can be mentally relived, fantasies about future meetings may occur, and a severe sadness and longing may be felt. Love always includes some level of attachment and this attachment to somebody may continue for the rest of one's life. In many cultures, people sing "I will love you until the end of time." In India, the Love between a man and a woman can be so strong that they take a vow to reincarnate for each other always. It is this vow that led to the disputed tradition of widow-burning *(sati)*, which was believed to ensure that the wife could become her dead husband's wife again in the next life.

The mood that is predominant in Bhakti Yoga (the yoga of spiritual devotion) strongly relates to Shringara, but also includes other Rasas such as Calmness and Wonder. The Love of the devotee is as real as in other types of Shringara, because the deity (including depictions such as pictures or sculptures) is seen as more real than anything else. The advanced *bhakta* (devotee) bypasses the addiction problem that is typical for other types of Shringara, because he or she feels that God is always around and available. Everything is God, so only unity is seen, even in the diversity of life. There is no need to look or long for God because God is felt everywhere. Nevertheless, the feeling of separation from God may create Sadness and the less advanced bhakti yogi may too strongly personalize his or her relationship with God and become overly jealous or fanatical toward others.

Bhakti Yoga is a very difficult path for the modern mind, because it requires the intellect to stop doubting God and Love without expectation. That is why in Bhakti Yoga the Bhava or mood of devotion must be maintained at every moment. Always keeping the place of worship clean and beautiful is a first but essential step in that direction.

Love in the Body

Butterflies in the stomach, goose bumps, sweating, trembling, and palpitations of the heart are some of the best-known symptoms of being in love. The very same symptoms can be felt in admiration of an object of art or natural beauty, or experienced through the devotion of the bhakti yogi.

The "chemistry" between lovers is today regarded as scientific fact. Science has, for example, recognized that endorphins (a group of neurotransmitters), our body's own opiate, are released upon eye contact between lovers, and that oxytocin triggers orgasms. Whether experienced through the sense of touch, as in sex, or through any of the other senses, or through thought processes alone, the body chemistry behind Shringara is always of a similar nature.

The science of Ayurveda regards Shringara as a rajasic Rasa that creates a lot of activity in body chemistry and is usually very healthy. The main element associated with Shringara is water and people who are kapha (mucus) dominated are the most able to Love and appreciate Beauty.

To be able to feel Love and admire the Beauty of life, our body chemistry must support it. If for example we eat too much junk food, our body chemistry will become so dull (tamasic) that we are unable to experience the finer feeling that Shringara really is. The body chemistry of adolescents strongly supports Shringara, making it their predominant Rasa. Spring is the time of the year when Shringara body chemistry is at its peak.

The basic problem of addiction in Shringara is expressed in body chemistry by the reduction in receptors for information molecules (see the discussion of drugs in chapter 3). Any "overdose" of enjoyment in Shringara will thus physically reduce our ability to enjoy. That is why enjoyment should be moderate and diversified, not excessive and obsessive. This is part of what "good taste" is all about.

The loss of reproductive fluid that occurs through sexual enjoyment is an important factor. The body stores the finer energies of prana, tejas, and especially ojas in the semen. As semen is the last dhatu or body constituent to be produced from the essence of food, which is Rasa as blood plasma, it has a very high concentration of the subtle energy that is Rasa (see chapter 17). Excessive sexual activity depletes this reserve of subtle energies and may produce negative emotions and a general lack of energy and health. The older we get, the more significant the effect.

Relationship to Other Rasas

Joy and Wonder are "friendly" Rasas that nourish Shringara when combined with it. Humor is much loved because it brings lightness and likewise people who create Humor are much loved. The smile of amusement and the smile of love are not very far apart. Joyful Humor is the Rasa that most often follows on Shringara.

The suspense and mystery that belong to the Wonder Rasa increase the feelings of Shringara if they indicate a special relationship between the people that are in love. For example, a lover might say that he dreamt about his beloved before they even met. Or a lady might feel that her lover is coming to visit her, even if she cannot yet see him.

Shringara, Joy, and Wonder form a very powerful trio, a guaranteed formula for attaining happiness. Likewise, in art, poetry, drama, and music, the feeling of Beauty can be enhanced by the addition of the sense of lightness that is typical of Joy and the sense of mystery and hidden meanings that is typical of Wonder.

Sadness, Courage, Anger, Fear, and Disgust are enemy Rasas of Shringara and can destroy the feeling when they are strong enough. Sadness is a passive, inward-turning emotion that may be helped by Love, but diminishes it, because Love is active, outward turning, and requires feedback. Courage is too focused on objectives and ideals to sustain Love. Even though heroes are loved and admired, love stories with heroes usually end in tragic drama. Heroes belong to society, not to any individual. Anger is regarded as the opposite of Love, while Disgust is the opposite of Beauty and good taste. Both reject Love and destroy Beauty. The Fear of losing Love may prevent it from growing or destroy it when it is already present.

Calmness is neutral in its relationship to Shringara; it is neither an enemy Rasa nor a friendly one. Shringara is active, while Calmness is inactive. Shringara can only be a friendly Rasa to Calmness in Bhakti Yoga, where decoration and ritual serve to focus and calm the mind, while Love for the deity brings humbleness to the ego, which is essential for attaining Calmness.

Mastering Love

To master Shringara we must first of all realize that Beauty is everywhere and is always there to be loved. Beauty is the divine nature of everything. If we cannot see that all-pervading Beauty, then some people and things become beautiful and lovable while others seem not. The fine and divine sense within that understands and admires Beauty must be used only in creation, not in evaluation. Everything can be made even more beautiful, but that understanding should not destroy the Beauty inherent in everything. Beauty is there to be enjoyed, not weighed. We must Love with admiration and admire with Love. The double meaning of the word Shringara—Beauty and Love—hides the main key to control it.

Second, every person and everything is capable of Love and of improvement, including oneself. Love and Beauty only need a little attention to be enhanced. They are divine qualities that only require some positive feedback to grow. Increasing Love and Beauty is about small and simple things, a touch here, a flower there, a smile, a little neatness, attention, and harmony. In some difficult cases, creating Love and Beauty may require the devotion and sacrifice that is the subject of so many dramatic stories, movies, and lives. But if we can maintain undoubting faith in the Love and Beauty that is inherent in everything, sooner than later they will come out radiantly. Beauty and Love should in any case be given without expectation of a reward.

Third, while Love and Beauty can be created without measure or restraint, they should be enjoyed with moderation and in diversity. The nature of our mind requires both to remain happy. The fulfillment of a desire removes the desire, making the hunt and moderate tasting much longer lasting than full consumption. Tasting, rather than eating, is the essence of the art of romance. Moreover, when we focus too much on a single object of enjoyment, the ego becomes too involved for happiness to remain. It is the nature of the ego to become attached through identification and since nothing in this world of illusion *(maya)* lasts forever, attachment leads to disappointment and from there to one of the enemy Rasas of Love.

Fourth, if we can remain as mere spectators, not personally involved in whatever is happening, and non-discriminating, then Beauty and Love can be enjoyed without measure. The person who loves everyone and everything is always in love. Whatever lovable person or thing goes away is automatically replaced by the next, which is equally lovable.

Couples should understand that attachment goes against the very nature of Shringara. While we may very well and beautifully choose a personal, long-term, and faithful relationship, it is important to accept that other relationships, of different kinds, need to be allowed and even stimulated. The lover who restrains the beloved from friendship with other people cannot expect love to last a lifetime. The nuclear family ideal is hardly a century old in the West and is already creating many problems in other cultures as well. While in many cultures monogamy was the rule, people often used to live together in large family houses where Love and Beauty could be enjoyed in much wider diversity. Spending time alone as a couple then was something rare and treasured, rather than an everyday bore. The divine game of hide and seek remains enjoyable only if it is never ending.

As Love and Beauty are essentially the same Rasa, Love should be enhanced by decoration and art, and vice versa. Love and love-making should be embedded in other enjoyments to be truly savored. Sex may be a natural urge, but it should not stand out like the salt or sugar in junk foods. Sexual enjoyment has the effect of a very powerful drug and thus one should beware of addiction and the over-consumption of vital energy. Only when it is diversified and moderated does sexual love remain interesting on the levels of body and mind, until at a later age people naturally and gradually lose interest in it. The Indian heritage is far from puritanical when it comes to sex, but it offers guidance about how sex can be enjoyed artfully. The fulfillment of this natural desire is quite all right if done in good taste or Rasa, which is explained in full detail in the Kama Sutra, India's great scripture on the art of Love.

Sexual desire belongs to the second chakra. If this chakra remains dissatisfied, it will block the opening of the higher chakras. If the sexual desire is really present, then only fulfilling it can exhaust it. After all, if all men and women were to remain celibate, how would saints be born? Sexual activity is most natural in the second stage of life, the *grihastha* or householder period (see chapter 22).

True Love and true Beauty are found on the inside of the beloved and are everlasting. If a person can see the divine in his or her beloved, then that Love will always remain. In India, women see their husbands as Krishna, Rama, or Shiva, while men see their wives as Radha, Sita, or Parvati. When men become gods and women goddesses, then Love truly becomes divine leela. Then the husband or wife is easy to Love without attachment and the roles of husband and wife become easy to play for eternity. Developing such an attitude is less difficult than it seems. In fact, when we admire the Beauty of the body and character of our husband or wife, we are really perceiving the god or goddess. We do not see the imperfections, and see only perfection, divinity. That is what being in love is all about. Problems in love start when we forget to ignore imperfections.

Another cause of problems in love and marriage is that physical and emotional attraction occur most naturally between two people who are rather different. While these differences thus lead to love marriages, they may cause severe problems later on when the two people become life partners who have to live and share everything together. As love thus makes lovers blind, Indian society still largely prefers arranged marriages, where parents analyze the compatibility of two people in marriage by analyzing their *varna* (caste in terms of basic interests in money, power, protection, charity, or spirituality), *vashia* (physiology and psychology), *nakshatra* (astrological constellations), *guna* (divine, human, and demonic tendencies), *dhinari* (age of the soul), and a large number of other aspects. While Indian parents do accept love marriages, they still feel the need to analyze these aspects of compatibility. Such intervention by parents may be unthinkable to Western youths, but even modern couples often benefit from having their compatibility for life partnership analyzed more rationally.

Marriages may also suffer when one or another or both of the partners are not really made for it. Some people remain eternal playboys and playgirls, or may be born saints that find little attraction in marriage.

The more traditional job division between the husband (who works outside of the house) and the wife (who works inside the house) assures that there is little need for discussion, as both have their domain in which they can feel confident, efficient, and valuable. While there is no real need to stick to such traditional job divisions between men and women, some more modern kind of job division may allow the couple to really enjoy their time together, rather than needing to have a practical agenda to discuss every time they meet.

Last but not least, by losing faith in the Divine, faith in marriage also is lost. When we stop seeing everything as divine will, then everything becomes a matter of individual choice and discrimination. Then life partners are ever scrutinized and easily discarded when found lacking.

The only truly permanent Love is that for God and God's creation: For never-changing consciousness and ever-changing energy, for Shiva and Shakti, soul *(purusha)* and primordial nature *(prakriti)*. Within this game of hide and seek, the pleasure lies in finding, the pain in not finding. When one Loves all, only pleasure remains.

To fully master Love, love the drop of consciousness that is in each and every soul and has all of the properties of the vast ocean of cosmic consciousness. Love your and our Self, whose nature is divine and in which resides all divine tendencies. Nurture the Love of Self and all and Love will be yours to enjoy forever, as it was never lost, but always around as our true nature, desire, purpose, and destiny.

Love Sadhana

Shringara Sadhana means that for a period of time you are ever tasteful, nice, sweet spoken, tender, and loving in deed, word, and thought. That means that not only must all enemy Rasas be kept out of your mind, but also that you should be completely focused on universal Love and Beauty only. This is not a matter of rationalization, but of true feeling.

The siddhi or power obtained when performing Shringara Sadhana for a prolonged period is *prapti* (attainment), the power to get whatever one wants. This power only comes if the sadhana is successful on the level of thought and if none of the enemy Rasas is felt, even for a very short period. A minute of Anger can eat the result of a one-year sadhana. It is generally not advisable to undertake Shringara Sadhana if you have not yet done sadhana of the enemy Rasas (see related chapters as well as chapter 15).

You may start doing Shringara Sadhana for a day now and then, just to increase your capability to feel this Rasa. Later it can be increased to one week, one month, or even longer, so that you really come to master Shringara. To fundamentally alter not only body chemistry but also your very being (up to the neural patterns, energy patterns, etc.) Shringara Sadhana of a year or more will be needed.

A minor version of Shringara Sadhana is to observe cleanliness and the aesthetic sense in your body, dress, and home at all times. Such Sadhana may not bring any high powers, but it certainly will increase your happiness and the quality of your relationships with others.

The true bhakti yogi performs a very pure Shringara Sadhana. Everything is God and God is Love and Beauty. If the sadhana can be maintained, the power of prapti will emerge.

Krishna: Deity of Love

Even though most Hindu deities are somehow associated with Love and Beauty, Krishna is the ruling deity of Shringara. As with every incarnation of Vishnu, the main purpose of the Krishna incarnation was to restore the balance of good and evil. He defeated the powerful demon Kansa and many of his minions. However, another purpose was just as important: The creation of the religion of Love.

As the story goes, the gods and high saints *(rishis)* complained to Vishnu that even though they were continuously concentrating on him and his name or mantra, they never could experience him in the flesh. So Vishnu invited them to incarnate as the gopis or milkmaids of Vrindavan during the time when he became Krishna. Foremost among the gopis was Radha, the incarnation of Lakshmi, Vishnu's spouse and Krishna's obvious favorite.

It so happened and young Krishna was adored by the gopis from the time he was a baby. The older he became, the more intense became their relationship. He was a divine flute-player and would play endless songs near the Yamuna River with all the gopis and his friends listening and many animals as well. Krishna is supposed to have been so beautiful that anybody who looked at him completely forgot about him- or herself. He was always beautifully dressed and adorned with the feathers of a peacock, another symbol of Shringara.

On one long-ago "Rasa Purnima"—a full-moon night in September when the sky becomes clear after the rainy season and the Moon is nearest to Earth and looks very big—Krishna invited the gopis for what is called the "Rasa Leela," the play of Rasa. Under that moonlit sky, Krishna danced with the gopis and fulfilled their desire for union with him. In order to be able to dance with every gopi, Krishna became as many bodies as there were gopis. The "Rasa Jatna" is an annual festival that still celebrates the "sports" of Krishna with the milkmaids of Vrindavan.

The adolescent or mature Rasa Leela that is often shown in art is only a fantasy of the artists and their customers. In fact, Krishna was only eight years old when he left Vrindavan to study in the ashram of the Rishi Sandeepani. Therefore, everything that happened between Krishna and Radha or Krishna and the gopis took place when he was a child. Krishna was very conscious of being Vishnu and the gopis were not ordinary women, but rather deities and realized beings that could experience leela in its purest form. Whatever happened on that "Rasa Leela" night can only have been very romantic and spiritual.

The Shringara Rasa between Krishna and the gopis is the divine play (leela) between reality (consciousness) and maya (illusion), purusha (soul) and prakriti (primordial nature), divinity and humanity. The gopis dance around Krishna as electrons dance around the nucleus of every atom, and as body molecules and energies dance around the chitta of every being.

Some of the most famous devotional songs about Krishna were composed by the former Rajput queen Meerabai, who beautifully sings of her love for Krishna, of her hope for union with Krishna, and of the pain of separation from Krishna. The songs of Meera also show that jealousy is an emotion related to Shringara, such as when she becomes jealous of Krishna's flute, which is allowed to touch his lips and into which he breathes the breath of life.

At a later age, as described in the Bhagavad Gita, Krishna creates the foundation for Bhakti Yoga, the yoga of devotion. His conversation on this subject with Arjuna during the great battle of Kurukshetra is world-famous. He explains how bhakti is the most direct method to experience the divine. All yoga rests on the foundation stone of true faith, true devotion, true bhakti. All forms literally become the deity, which in turn becomes the devotee. Acceptance of leela or divine play as our basic nature gives devotion to life itself. Knowledge makes a wise person, who still has to travel a long way to reach God. Devotion makes a divine child, ever surrounded by the benevolent protection of the deity in myriad names and forms.

SHRINGARA RASA SUMMARY

Basic Rasa	Love
Sub-Rasas	Beauty, Admiration, Aesthetic Sentiment, Devotion
Dominant Element	Water
Dominant Dosha	Kapha
Dominant Guna	Rajas
Dominant Kosha	Mind (Manomaya Kosha)
Friendly Rasas	Joy, Wonder
Enemy Rasas	Sadness, Disgust, Anger, Courage, Fear
Neutral Rasas	Calmness
Rasa Produced	Joy
Key for Mastering	Love in good taste but without discrimination
Siddhi	Prapti (attainment)
Deity	Krishna

6

Hasya: Joy

Humor reveals the true nature of life.

The Basis of Joy

The purest Hasya is a Joy that comes from within for no apparent reason, and is not linked to actions or events. Yogis call it *ahladini shakti* or "the power of Joy." Ahladini shakti may also come when we feel that God or life is kind. It is found sometimes in crazy people and often in children and young people. This Hasya is a divine Rasa, an expression of divine bliss, symbolized by Radha, the favorite of Krishna.

Humor—the second significant meaning of Hasya—is, however, linked to particular situations. The favorite subject of Humor is *maya,* the illusionary aspect of the universe, the eternal play of opposites that is never the ultimate truth but merely a reflection of truth. In a joke, something becomes a reason for laughter because it demonstrates the futility of attaching too much importance to what is actually an illusion. There is nothing funny about a person who stumbles, except if they were previously showing a lot of pride. Laughing at our worries means we understand that the future can bring anything: It may bring what we fear, or its opposite, or even something completely unexpected.

Basically, Humor takes the seriousness out of life, and what else is this seriousness but a hanging on to our illusionary roles and games, against all evidence? The art of Humor is to reveal the opposite forces that are at work in whatever happens.

The subject of Humor also depends on the level of consciousness. For people who mostly reside in the first chakra, the favorite themes are basic fears and bodily functions. They laugh about defecation, burping, grave accidents, horror scenes, and so on. For those who primarily reside in the second chakra, the favorite subjects are sex, sensuality, and relationships. For third chakra people, the egos of others are the favorite object of laughter, such as when someone fails to be what they pretend or want to be. For fourth chakra people, love, affection, and devotion are the topics of the best jokes. For fifth chakra people, knowledge or its absence is the preferred subject. For sixth chakra people, it becomes maya itself.

The ego is a highly popular object of Humor in general. Those who can make fun of themselves are clowns. It is the mind that sees the joke. If the ego accepts the joke, even a joke on itself, laughter comes. The minute the intellect starts intervening, real Humor is impossible. Then innocent laughter becomes satire or sarcasm.

Even saints need and have Joy. Laughter is very relaxing. In India, people believe that if the sage Narada, who represents pure wisdom, stayed in one place for more than forty-five minutes, the world would end. We can take only so much wisdom; after that some Humor is needed.

When life seems like hell, laughter brings us immediately back to Earth if not to heaven. With laughter, life on Earth becomes satisfying enough. Laughter is highly infectious, which makes funny people very popular. Entertainment must always have some element of Humor: a circus or a play must always have a clown or a fool.

Some people are world famous for their mastery of Humor, such as Laurel and Hardy, Charlie Chaplin, Patch Adams, Louis De Funes, and many more.

Sub-Rasas of Joy

The main sub-Rasas of Hasya are satire and sarcasm, the latter being even more a mixture with the Rasas of Anger or Disgust than the former. They involve the intellect and as such are not real Joy or Humor, which are innocent. Such combinations of Rasas can only be short-lived.

Teasing is a mild form of satire. There is nothing wrong with some teasing between friends. The monkey that is our mind enjoys being pulled by the tail—it is just another reason for jumping around. As long as we know that the ego of the person that is the object of the joke can take it, the humor can remain relatively pure. Usually it is also very instructive, a friendly way of pointing out some fault to provide an opportunity for improvement.

Satire has a similar use in a broader social context. The fool can say things to the king that otherwise might have been left unsaid. Thus, satire has had a great role to play throughout history.

Joy in the Body

The Hasya Rasa is dominated by the fire element and is rajasic. Laughter brings heat to the entire body, particularly to the head and ears. When we laugh, we have a tendency to tense the muscles at the height of the third chakra, which is also dominated by the fire element. Pitta dominated people easily laugh.

Various neurochemicals play a role in the effects of Joy. Generally, it increases the endorphins and serotonin, while reducing dopamine, norepinephrine, and cortisol.

Hasya is very healthy and rejuvenating. It reduces tension, Anger, Fear, or depression and helps in digestion. Indian people have the healthy habit of always telling jokes after a meal. The fire element produced aids the digestive fire. Humor and Joy also improve our immunity against infections and strengthen our cardiovascular system.

Relationship to Other Rasas

Love is the companion Rasa of Hasya and the purest Joy is experienced with those we Love. Joy creates Love and vice versa. Together, they are unbeatable.

The Rasa of Wonder is also friendly to Hasya, which means that a joke becomes even stronger when an element of mystery is included. Wonder is also fire-dominated and creates a tension, which when released increases the power of Humor. Humor is a nice way to deal with the mystery of life.

Sadness or pity, Disgust, and Fear are the enemy Rasas of Joy. If they are powerful enough, they can destroy Joy. Joy is an enemy Rasa to Sadness and Fear, but neutral toward Disgust (which can only be countered by Shringara). Sadness is the opposite Rasa of Joy.

While Anger is neutral to Joy, Joy is an enemy Rasa to Anger. Humor and Anger may coexist in satire or sarcasm, but they form a dangerous and impure combination that may lead to more Anger and Disgust. The famous epic war of the Mahabharata was started by the disrespectful joke Draupadi made to Duryodhana about the blindness of his father.

In conclusion, Joy or Humor is a very powerful tool against Sadness, Fear, and Anger. Always remember the very powerful mantra that solves any problem:

OM NO PROBLEM, OM NO PROBLEM, OM NO
PROBLEM, OM NO PROBLEM . . .

Calmness and Courage are neutral to Joy, while Joy is an enemy Rasa to Calmness. Inactivity does not disturb activity, but activity disturbs inactivity.

Pure Joy is endless and creates only more Joy.

Mastering Joy

While Joy can be consciously inhibited, we cannot consciously produce laughter. It is very difficult to laugh on command or to fake laughter convincingly. Hasya depends not so much on the occasion, but on the presence of ahladini shakti, joy energy, in the body. Natural Joy is the reward for seeing the Beauty of life.

This energy is very much present in children and adolescents, who can laugh without end for no apparent reason. As we grow older, natural laughter gets easily lost because of changes in body chemistry and cultural inhibitions. All we can do to increase the occurrence of Hasya in life is to love life and others, release tensions, maintain a healthy body and attitude to life, and be uninhibitedly open to laughter when it comes. By understanding the illusionary nature of creation, we also see the Beauty and Love inherent in life. Then God always seems kind, whatever happens, and the energy of Joy remains.

Producing Hasya in others requires talent, care, and discipline, along with a perfect sense of good taste (Shringara). Laughter is highly infectious, so if we can make one person laugh, others will easily follow. This effect is so strong that when two people start laughing, others often easily join in, even if they do not know the reason for it. The best way to produce Hasya in oneself is to create it in others. Harish Johari was a real master of that game. Next to his love and wisdom, his humor was certainly one of the reasons for the popularity of his classes.

When it comes, inner Humor is very valuable and should certainly not be inhibited, even if others might feel it strange to see somebody laugh because of some "inside" joke.

Joy Sadhana

The sadhana of Hasya consists of laughing without end, of fasting on Joy and Humor only. This is obviously a very hard sadhana that is not easily accepted by others and requires an enormous amount of self-control. It is so easy to become serious and even that is a joke. To see the Humor of any situation requires a deep understanding of the illusionary nature of the universe.

Because this sadhana is so difficult, it is often performed in a reduced form. Harish Johari gave the example of a professor who was doing a lifelong Humor Sadhana. While teaching he would be very serious, but when not performing that duty, he would express only ridicule and laughter. There are still people in India who laugh all the time, without any concern about the impressions they make upon others. They are called *mukta*, liberated. Most people think they are crazy and some may well be, while others are not. It is hard to tell the difference since no serious word is ever uttered.

To experience how difficult this sadhana is, try it just for an hour or so. To kill any serious thought is a very difficult discipline, because both mind and intellect will continuously try to make the ego believe that something or other is threatening, unfair, or whatever, and in need of serious attention. To do this sadhana for a full day is a very good exercise that will confront us with our innermost worries and desires. With Hasya Sadhana, there is no longer a need to continue falling down cliffs in order to truly understand that Humor is the only way up. Once the sadhana is successful for a short period, it may be a little difficult to stop it.

The siddhi obtained through Hasya Sadhana is called *vashitva* (popularity), the power to control others by thought alone.

Little Krishna: The Deity of Joy

Krishna is the ruling deity of both Shringara and Hasya, because they are companion Rasas. The association with Hasya also comes through Radha, who is the personification of ahladini shakti.

Krishna is very famous for teasing the gopis and his foster-mother Yashoda when he was a child. One day he had taken some mud in his mouth, but he denied it; to prove that he had not done it, he told Yashoda to look into his mouth. When she looked, she saw the entire universe. Krishna was known for stealing and throwing butter and milk and even for stealing the clothes of the milkmaids when they took a bath in the river. When they were ashamed to come out naked, he reminded them of their true nature and of their devotion to him.

Little Krishna was not just teasing purely for the fun of it. He wanted to destroy the ignorance of his devotees, teaching them not to be attached to matter and forms and to focus only on him. The Humor created by Krishna thus shows the illusionary nature of maya and results in feelings of Wonder and Love.

HASYA RASA SUMMARY

Basic Rasa	Joy
Sub-Rasas	Humor, Satire, Sarcasm
Dominant Element	Fire
Dominant Dosha	Pitta
Dominant Guna	Rajas
Dominant Kosha	Mind (Manomaya Kosha)
Friendly Rasas	Love, Wonder
Enemy Rasas	Sadness, Disgust, Fear
Neutral Rasas	Calmness, Courage, Anger
Rasa Produced	Joy
Key for Mastering	Make others see the beauty of the illusion of life
Siddhi	Vashitva (popularity)
Deity	Little Krishna

7

Adbhuta: Wonder

The grandest crime of science is to limit truth
to its own limited understanding.

The Basis of Wonder

From the dawn of civilization, human beings have tried to understand everything and are still trying. The feeling of Wonder comes when we recognize our own ignorance. When a wonderful thing happens, the intellect is overwhelmed, unable to fully understand it, the mind is completely immersed in the feeling of Wonder, and the ego surrenders to it.

Wonder is enjoyable because it brings the promise of learning. When we understand that there are things that we do not understand, it makes life beautiful and exciting, full of wonders to explore, full of opportunity for new understanding and personal growth. Life without some mystery is terribly boring and dull; the older we get, the more we understand, and the more important it becomes to experience wonderful things.

Wonder comes at the beginning of the spiritual journey, the journey to find real truth and solve the mystery of life. However much we may come to know, part of the mystery of life will always remain unknown, so the Adbhuta Rasa will always remain and people will continue to start on the spiritual path because of it. New religions are often supported by miracles.

Mystery is only ignorance—the moment we know what is happening and how, the Adbhuta Rasa disappears. Modern science declares that it understands virtually everything and what it cannot explain is simply said to be nonexistent by definition. It continues to promote this attitude in spite of the fact that it is continuously researching and understanding new things. It does so with complete disregard for the emotional health of people who need the feeling of Wonder. To discard that which one cannot understand is a game of the ego of the scientists, nothing more.

Even though science understands a lot, the birth of a child or the growth of a seed into a tree remain great mysteries. The Big Bang and the tiny atoms and energies of which we are made are mysterious. Quantum physics shows that reality is not concrete at all and that deterministic scientific laws are no more than mathematics of probability. What happens to us after death is another of the great mysteries; the creator of all the marvelous and complex things that science comes to understand is the biggest mystery of all.

Despite the impact of Western science, Adbhuta is still a very popular Rasa. Everybody desires to live through something that is truly miraculous, unpredictable, unimaginable, and wonderful. Part of the purpose of the ancient stories of all cultures is to create Wonder and thus reduce the ego. Even today we see an increase in the popularity of this Rasa, for example in the popularity of books, movies, and games that deal with fantasy and magic, such as the Harry Potter adventures or the Lord of the Rings saga. The whole of humanity is waiting for something really mysterious to happen, because it is not agreeable to know everything.

Real saints that can do real magic sometimes appear to show humankind that what we register through sense perception is not truth; they attempt to break the inflated egos of modern humans and science. Unfortunately, fake saints also create tricky magic that causes a lot of damage to the image of real saints. The real saint is most often very careful and discriminating in demonstrating special powers, because such powers are not to be used lightly. They can draw attention that may destroy his peace and attract greedy people. A true saint also recognizes that blind faith has caused faith in general to get a bad image and has been a main factor in creating the current dominance of rationalism and skepticism.

The truth is that nothing and everything is magical, depending on one's understanding. Through yogic science, things become possible that are miracles to people who do not understand this science. As everything is One, so everything can become anything—that is the true nature of every yogic miracle. The fact that magicians are able to reproduce those effects by performing tricks is no proof of the contrary.

The powers that a yogi may achieve through sadhana are not very important in themselves. The reward of sadhana goes far beyond them. Still, to some spiritual students the possibility of attaining them may be an extra motivation as well as a confirmation of the true divinity of life and of the value of the chosen spiritual path. Spiritual stories as well as the personal witnessing of spiritual powers transport us from purely physical perception to the world beyond maya, the illusion of diversity in the universe.

Sub-Rasas of Wonder

There are two kinds of Wonder. The first type of Wonder is felt when we experience something that we do not understand, along with knowing that a rational explanation is available. For example, this Wonder is felt when we attend a magic show and we know that what is seen is just a trick, but we still don't understand it. Another example is when we witness a machine being brought near Saturn to photograph its rings, without understanding much of the technologies behind it, but still knowing that there is no magic involved. In this type of Wonder, the ego feels only slightly threatened and the feeling most often results in laughter and in admiration for the skill of the magician or whoever is accomplishing something remarkable or difficult.

The second and much stronger type of Wonder comes when we are confronted with something so miraculous that we cannot possibly expect to understand it. It occurs when we are faced with some miraculous spiritual experience, such as a touch of the divine in meditation, a demonstration of supernatural powers by real saints, or a near-death experience. Certainly also scientists may experience it when their study reveals to them the endless complexity of this universe or of the object of their study. This type of Wonder completely subdues the ego, at least for a time, and leads us to accept our ignorance and basic insignificance. It is a first step toward wisdom.

Wonder in the Body

Wonder is dominated by the fire element; the feeling will heat up the entire body. It is rajasic in nature and pitta dominated. The neurochemicals involved remain a mystery to modern science, as far as can be detected in scientific literature.

Relationship to Other Rasas

As previously mentioned, the feeling of Wonder is helpful to the Rasas of Love and Joy. Both the feelings of Love and the natural laughter of real Joy may produce some Wonder as well, because they bring a revelation that is difficult to fully understand or describe. This revelation involves the divine and, at the same time, illusionary nature of existence. Yet both Love and Joy are neutral to Wonder, because when something truly wonderful happens, the Love of other people experiencing it or the pure Joy that they might feel about it will have little effect on one's own feeling. Courage and Disgust are also neutral to Wonder, since neither requires an explanation. Calmness also is neutral. Anger is an enemy Rasa to Wonder, as an angry person is so ego-centered that he or she may not notice anything else, wonderful or not.

Fear however is a friendly Rasa to Adbhuta, because in both the ego is subdued. That which we do not understand always becomes a little fearsome. This is also part of the explanation for the unpopularity of the Wonder Rasa among scientists and rationalists. To deny existence to anything that one does not understand or cannot control is truly a cowardly reaction, often found in children. The feeling of Wonder is thus destroyed in order to reduce Fear. To the one who is fearless, everything is wonderful because one allows oneself to experience it that way.

Sadness also is a friendly Rasa to Wonder, because Sadness subdues the ego and because the cause of Sadness is often something hard to understand. When something sad happens, the people who are sad because of it always wonder why it happened, how it could happen, why it happened to them, and so on.

The Rasa most often produced through Wonder is the Joy that life is wonderful and exciting.

Mastering Wonder

Wonder is not a Rasa that we can create by will, even though it can be willfully denied. The key to Wonder is to remain open-minded toward the miracle of life, which can be experienced in everything. When something happens that we do not immediately understand, it is important to taste that feeling and let it have its desirable effect on the ego, before giving in to the desire to find out what has taken place. This is true both for a box of disappearing chocolates (probably simply plundered by children), as well as for any higher miracles that we may be fortunate enough to witness.

Unfortunately, tricky people exist as well as true miracles, so we have to judge carefully. When faced with a person demonstrating what seems like real power, we have to remember that the miracles witnessed are no more important than the more obvious miracles that can be witnessed everywhere anytime. A budding flower is a miracle, whether the flower is taking its time naturally or whether it happens more rapidly in the hands of a saint. The real value of a saint must be measured by other means, such as the ability to enhance the quality of meditation of people nearby or by the levels of control needed to maintain a saintly life. With true saints, both observations provide enough opportunity for very strong feelings of motivating Wonder.

Maya or illusion exists only because of ignorance. Divine leela could not be experienced without it. We need to find the right balance between blind faith and pedantry. Seeking out the less obvious miracles is a favorite past time for many, but there is no real need to fly to the Moon since we are already in space.

Wonder Sadhana

The highest Wonder Sadhana means to completely refrain from the idea of understanding anything, to be always conscious of our ignorance. Whatever happens is a miracle by definition and it is useless to wonder about the why and how. Nothing can be understood; no explanation can be taken for granted; only astonishment is suitable.

This sadhana is very difficult, because it is difficult to decide to engage in an action without understanding what the result might be. Action must then truly be taken without any expectation of gain. To do this sadhana you have to realize that whatever happens, happens, and then just follow the flow of life without choosing any particular direction. When you feel hungry, you can try to see if eating solves the problem. The ever-inquiring mind and especially the ever-judging intellect must be kept quiet. Truly, this is a sadhana for advanced yogis only.

A less difficult form of Wonder Sadhana consists of not denying that which you do not understand. You can make a distinction between that which you think you understand and that which you do not, but without taking a position toward that which is beyond your understanding. The miraculous nature of the world should never be denied.

The power obtained when performing true Wonder Sadhana is the power of *laghima* or lightness. This power allows one to become so light that one can fly.

Brahma: The Deity of Wonder

Creation is the greatest mystery, so Brahma—the creator within the Hindu trinity of Brahma, Vishnu (the preserver), and Shiva (the destroyer)—is the ruling deity of the Wonder Rasa. Brahma is also seen as the ruling deity of this Rasa because the Vedas, four books containing all of the sacred mysteries of Hinduism, sprang from his four heads. His name also relates to Brahman, the universal spirit that is an even greater mystery than creation itself. He is thus also related to the Brahmins, the caste of priests that are supposed to know Brahman and preserve the mysteries. In many Hindu epics, other gods turn to Brahma whenever something goes wrong and expect him to perform a miracle to solve it.

On numerous occasions throughout Hindu mythology, Brahma also causes problems by granting special powers to demons that worship him. The best known among them is Ravana, who was able to conquer all the worlds and heavens because of his special powers until Vishnu incarnated as Rama to stop him. Although the use of special powers can evoke Wonder, it is inferior to the Wonder of divine creation itself. These stories about Brahma are a warning not to confuse special powers with divinity and to bestow and use them carefully.

ADBHUTA RASA SUMMARY

Basic Rasa	Wonder
Sub-Rasas	Curiosity, Astonishment
Dominant Element	Fire
Dominant Dosha	Pitta
Dominant Guna	Rajas
Dominant Kosha	Mind (Manomaya Kosha)
Friendly Rasas	Fear, Sadness
Enemy Rasas	Anger
Neutral Rasas	Calmness, Courage, Love, Joy, Disgust
Rasa Produced	Joy
Key for Mastering	Humbly accept the mystery of normality
Siddhi	Laghima (lightness)
Deity	Brahma

8

Shanta: Calmness

*Real peace comes in meditation to the one
who is free of debt and desire.*

The Basis of Calmness

The Shanta Rasa is the Rasa of preference for saints, yogis, and sadhus. Real Shanta exists only in *samadhi,* a state of super-consciousness that is the final stage of any yoga. For true Calmness, body, mind, ego, and intellect must become perfectly still. The I-consciousness and the supreme consciousness become one, while even the most essential bodily functions such as breathing come to a halt.

The pure state of Calmness is impossible to describe except by negation, because in pure Calmness there are no words left. Even if only the memory of "who I am" remains, then with me all my problems and my world also remain and Shanta becomes impossible.

For a long time, Shanta was not even regarded as a Rasa by the Indian tradition because it is without emotion, ni-rasa. It was not included in the Natya Shastra, the overview of dramatic art written by Bharata in the fourth or fifth century. It was only in the eleventh century that Abhinavagupta noted it as the ninth Rasa.

Everybody longs for real peace of mind, though only a few saints really attain it. Calmness is very popular but rare, while Anger is very unpopular but common. In modern society, the Shanta Rasa has become more and more rare and unpopular, while in ancient Indian society it was regarded as the highest state of being. Even if not many could attain it, those who tried were held in high regard. Today, many people regard saints as people who are simply doing nothing. What they do not understand is how difficult and rewarding doing nothing really is.

Sub-Rasas of Calmness

Rest and exhaustion are both sub-Rasas of Calmness. In deep sleep, everybody attains Shanta. While the mind remains very active in the dream state, in deep sleep, everybody loses the I-consciousness and thus peace is attained. That state of complete rest is extremely important for the revitalization of both body and mind, so the duration and depth of deep sleep is extremely important for attaining a more peaceful mind and life. Not sleeping for several days can cause people to become crazy for the rest of their lives (for more about sleep, see chapter 18).

Taking a break now and then is very important too, even though it is not real Shanta because mind, body, and ego remain active. Relaxation of any kind, preferably including the reduction and purification of sensory input, should be a daily habit and will improve the depth and duration of deep sleep. All regular meditation practices have this result.

Hard physical labor or extreme mental activity may also lead to a kind of Calmness. There are also various kinds of non-yogic states of extreme absorption (samadhi), such as coma, vision, stupor, and so on. In these states, one completely forgets oneself by being completely absorbed in something that is not cosmic consciousness, but has a more rajasic or tamasic nature.

Calmness in the Body

In yogic samadhi, all movement of the body stops and even the bodily functions that are auto-regulated by the brain stem stop or become extremely slow. Being able to stop their breath and heartbeat (without dying) is one of the feats of wonder with which yogis have been able to surprise modern scientists on numerous occasions. Some of them have, for example, been submerged in water or put in an airtight container for over twenty-four hours.

The element of the Shanta Rasa is air, which is normally associated with the extreme activity that occurs in Fear, the only other air-dominated Rasa. If the vata dosha (which contains the elements air and akasha) is disturbed, peace of mind is not possible because the vata dosha creates restlessness. In Shanta, the air element becomes pure prana, charged with negative ions. Air is neutral, even though it may carry various energies and traces of other elements. Inner peace is found at the level of the fourth chakra, the seat of the soul, which is dominated by the air element as well.

The breathing exercises taught to women for use during childbirth increase the body's endorphin levels. This natural body-morphine reduces pain as well as improves inner peace by enhancing contentment. Slowing down the breath slows down the heartbeat and reduces adrenaline production. Shallow and rapid breathing, on the contrary, creates nervousness. Breathing in Shanta is slow and deep, while in Fear it is rapid and shallow.

The Calmness Rasa is sattvic, while exhaustion or deep sleep is tamasic in nature. The gentle light of the sattva guna is very peace-giving and associated with the goddess Lakshmi.

Relationship to Other Rasas

Calmness has no friendly Rasas, with the exception of Karuna as Compassion. Shanta can tolerate universal Compassion, as taught by Buddha. Real Compassion can be a good motivation for exercising Shanta, because Compassion focuses not on the suffering but on the delusion of suffering, which can only be broken through detachment (see chapter 11). Karuna as personal Sadness, however, can be very disturbing to one's peace of mind. It is also possible to be so struck by grief that the mind, ego, and intellect simply shut down and one becomes unable to think or talk. This is an inferior kind of Calmness that is dominated by tamas and not by sattva.

Calmness is especially disturbed by those Rasas in which the ego becomes very important: Anger, Fear, Courage, and Love. But an exception can be seen in the Shringara of the bhakti yogi whose universal Love brings peace instead of destroying it (see chapter 5). Joy is also an enemy Rasa to Calmness, because it is too rajasic, though it does bring a lightness that can produce some peace. Disgust and Wonder are neutral to Calmness, because they both produce little ego-sense.

Because Calmness is ni-rasa, without Rasa, it is the only Rasa that can be mixed with any other Rasa. The result will not be pure Calmness, but a more peaceful form of the other Rasa. We can be calmly in love or calmly joyful. Some people are calmer than others even in Sadness or Anger. Maintaining a certain level of Calmness through regular relaxation and meditation increases our ability to master the other Rasas.

Periods of Calmness are mostly followed by Sadness because at that time we see most clearly how we are trapped in maya.

Mastering Calmness

Even if we feel that we are not enlightened, we can always give it our best shot. The main way to induce Calmness is through meditation practices, combined with keeping a balance between needs and desires. Desires are many, while needs are few. That which makes a saint so special is precisely the withdrawal from worldly desires. In order to attain Shanta, we should not cater to our desires that can buffet us about like the restless waves of the ocean. When we focus on what we truly need, then the winds of desire do not create any ripples on the surface of the pond.

This is supported by following our dharma, the code of conduct that best suits our place in society and our path to liberation. Doing so helps us to exhaust the effects of karma, the law of cause and effect by which we enjoy or suffer the results of past actions.

Following our dharma first of all means to pay our debts. The Indian tradition categorizes these debts into three kinds: debts to ancestors, debts to the universe, and debts to the teacher. Paying these three debts will provide a person with the satisfaction needed to attain real peace.

Clearing the debt to the ancestors means that, like them, we procreate and take care of one or more children. If our ancestors had not undertaken that charge, we would not be around. Some highly evolved souls might not need to pay this debt and may choose the path of a celibate yogi at a very early age. But most people do; only by paying this debt do they feel satisfied and able to properly meditate. Having children is also a great way to learn to set the ego and its desires aside. If the children are not happy, the parents won't be happy either.

Paying the debt to the universe means taking care of everything around us in gratitude for all we have been given by God and the universe. We cannot attain peace in meditation if we have neglected our responsibilities toward those who depend on us, whether they are friends or family, animals, or the environment that surrounds us.

Paying the debt to the teacher has nothing to do with paying the teacher for giving classes. Whether or not a spiritual teacher is paid depends on the situation of both teacher and student. The real debt owed to the teacher is that of passing on the teaching to others. Every student in turn has to become a teacher and pass on the teaching, preferably by adding his or her own experience to it. Those that keep the knowledge to themselves and dislike sharing it with others will not attain any real peace.

Another aspect of following dharma is to fulfill those desires that bring one to a higher state of being. It may be necessary even to fulfill some rather selfish desires in order to feel satisfied. As long as they do not become addictions, this is a very natural process of spiritual evolution in which desires are exhausted through fulfillment. Still, fulfilling such personal desires does not directly produce Shanta, because when one desire is fulfilled, another will emerge. Real satisfaction comes by fulfilling desires related to the well-being of others or related to sadhana, which is a part of paying our debt to the universe. Whether it involves strict yogic disciplines, simple fasting exercises, or Rasa Sadhana, the satisfaction that comes from following such disciplines removes the inner struggle. And by fulfilling these universal and spiritual desires our karma is also exhausted.

Only in this way do we become ready to practice real meditation. Then we can really learn to control our mind and the senses, the ego, and the intellect through various yogic paths, traditions, and practices (see chapter 22). Once a yogi has experienced real samadhi, he or she can always remain in Shanta by recalling it.

A very efficient tool to become calmer at any time is to temporarily hold the breath. Whenever we feel too excited or nervous, we should breathe in deeply and hold the breath as long as possible, while still reserving enough time to breath out slowly.

Calmness Sadhana

Real Calmness Sadhana can only be achieved by the yogi who has attained samadhi at least once. Such a person will remain so calm at all times that the Calmness will express itself around him or her, even in wild animals. The siddhi obtained by Shanta Sadhana is *anima,* the power to become smaller than an atom (atomicity).

For those who have not yet experienced samadhi, pure Shanta Sadhana is not possible, but everybody can exercise various levels of Shanta. By food fasting, Calmness of the digestive tract is obtained, and by speech fasting, we gain Calmness in communication. By doing yoga postures (asana), Calmness in posture is gained, while the practice of pranayama (conscious breath control), produces Calmness in breathing.

Vishnu: The Deity of Calmness

Vishnu is the preserver of creation and the ruling deity of the Shanta Rasa. He is always at peace. Even when incarnated in numerous forms he always remains an example of contentment and Shanta. He is always available as a preserver and protector, so he never sleeps. If we help

Vishnu in the preservation of the universe, we will experience his peace and may grant others fearlessness like Vishnu does.

SHANTA RASA SUMMARY

Basic Rasa	Calmness
Sub-Rasas	Rest, Exhaustion
Dominant Element	Air
Dominant Dosha	Vata
Dominant Guna	Sattva
Dominant Kosha	Chitta (Anandamaya Kosha)
Friendly Rasas	Sadness (as Compassion)
Enemy Rasas	Anger, Love, Joy, Fear, Courage
Neutral Rasas	Disgust, Wonder
Rasa Produced	Sadness
Key for Mastering	Meditate and pay your debts while reducing needs to a minimum
Siddhi	Anima (atomicity)
Deity	Vishnu

9

Raudra: Anger

With the help of all divine energies inside,
Anger can be easily defeated.

The Basis of Anger

When expectations are not fulfilled, the ego may feel that it has been neglected or treated incorrectly; this forms the basis for Anger. In Anger, the ego becomes extremely dominant. The mind follows the ego, though its attention may wander. The intellect may try to give soothing advice, but if overruled by the ego it will supply information that supports the Anger, such as the memory of earlier unfulfilled expectations.

The Anger that is based on the first chakra is caused by expectations that relate to insecurity. That Anger can become very violent, because it involves Fear. Anger in the second chakra is caused by unfulfilled sensory desires. In the third chakra, it is caused when people do not give us the respect that we expect.

Anger is the first of the Rasas that is regarded as demonic rather than divine. The divine and demonic energies have one father (Kashyapa Rishi) but two mothers (Diti and Aditi). Aditi gave birth to all of the divine beings *(devas)* and Diti gave birth to all of the demonic beings *(daitias, danavas,* and *rakshasas)*. The divine beings only give while demons only take. Human beings who only take, such as criminals, are ever angry, like demons or rakshasas. Those who only give are always peaceful, like gods or saints. In most people there is a mixture of demonic and divine, Anger and Calmness.

However, all religions have created one or many angry gods or have stories in which gods become angry. For example, when the head of her son Ganesha was cut off, Parvati demonstrated the power of all women. From her third eye all forms of the Devi or Mother Goddess, including the ferocious Kali and Durga, came forth in Anger to avenge her son. Such stories remind us of the power of Anger and that Anger can be constructive if it is instructive, such as the Anger of a mother toward her child, a teacher toward a student, a king toward his subjects, a friend toward a friend. In society, Anger is functional for administrators or anybody with a leading role. The fear of Anger and the resulting penalty makes people behave.

Some people harbor Anger over one particular subject all of their lives. The repetition of angry thoughts can work like a mantra that over time comes to dominate one's entire being. Similarly societies may keep Anger over generations, such as in the vendetta blood feuds for which Sicilian families are well known, or in the wars that have existed between some countries over the centuries.

Sub-Rasas of Anger

Irritation is a mild form of Anger, often related to the pressure that one suffers because of the expectations of others. Nervousness and stress may involve irritation, but belong more to the Fear Rasa. As Fear and Anger are friendly Rasas, these sub-Rasas contain both. A stressed, nervous person shifts between worry and irritation, depending on circumstance.

Violence is a sub-Rasa of Anger only if it happens in Anger. The Disgust Rasa may also cause violent behavior. Some violence may not relate to any Rasa at all, but might for example be based on greed or duty.

Anger in the Body

In Anger, the eyes are opened wide, while in Calmness the eyes are closed. Eyes can express more Anger than words. Anger can cause the jaw, the hands, or the whole body to become tight and tense. The entire body becomes hot, particularly the hands. The breathing pattern becomes fast and shallow and the sounds become harsh and loud. An angry person changes the entire environment and may affect the breathing pattern of others even if they are not involved in the subject of the Anger.

Anger is obviously rajasic and the element of the Anger Rasa is fire. Pitta dominated people are easier to anger than others. Anger can be a purifier that cleans negative emotional patterns. The burning yogic fire that comes out of the third eye of Shiva and of saints such as Vashista or Kapila is also caused by Anger. However, Anger is only beneficial for a very short time, when it burns the toxins created by dissatisfaction and irritation.

If Anger persists for some time, its fire starts eating the system from within, creating mental and bodily diseases. The fire of Anger disturbs pitta and makes the body chemistry become more acidic. This causes problems in joints and muscles, destroys the eyesight, causes cardiovascular disturbances such as heart attacks, and brings illness to the digestive and nervous systems.

Relationship to Other Rasas

Fear and Anger are friendly Rasas that easily go together. Fear may create Anger through the feeling of helplessness. At the heart of Anger may lie the Fear that injustice represents a precedent for further injustice. Then Anger becomes a preventive measure.

Joy, Love, and Wonder are enemy Rasas of Anger. Joy or Humor relaxes and removes the seriousness of Anger and the clouding caused by maya. Love offers an apology and that may satisfy the ego so much that it gives up the Anger. Wonder makes the ego become very small so that Anger is no longer possible.

Anger and Calmness are opposites because in Anger the ego becomes extremely powerful, while in Calmness it has to go. Nevertheless,

Calmness is neutral to Anger because it remains unnoticed by the angry person. On the contrary, one minute of Anger can eat the peace produced by one year of yoga.

Courage is also neutral to Anger. Courage can be supported by Anger but Anger does not need it and is not reduced by it.

Disgust contains a kind of Anger that is directed at everything, including oneself. In real Anger, the ego is so inflated that it does not tolerate Disgust toward it. The angry person sees no fault in him- or herself. Neither, however, does an angry person condemn Disgust in others, so the relationship is neutral.

In Anger, Compassion or Sadness only becomes an option after the fire has burned itself out. Karuna is the Rasa produced most often following Anger, but mostly as Sadness.

Mastering Anger

When Anger comes, there are basically three healthy ways to deal with it. The best way is to dissolve the Anger the moment it arises, by analyzing the unfulfilled expectation that lies at the basis of it, then shifting to one or more of its enemy Rasas—Joy, Love, or Wonder—if needed, followed by some purification of body chemistry. The second best option is to address the circumstances of the Anger in a non-violent way, if we feel that it is our duty or dharma to counter an injustice. The third best option is to play a role of being angry toward the person who is misbehaving, so that he or she gains a natural understanding that an important line has been crossed. Suppressing Anger is never an option, because it will continue to simmer inside.

The Anger expressed by one person can turn another person's Anger into Fear, as a child's Anger can disappear when it is faced with the Anger of the father or mother. However it is best both for the child and the parents if Anger can be acted without being felt, with the parents playing their appropriate role in the game of life. If that role requires punishment, so be it, as long as the punishment is not given to satisfy the parents' Anger. A child is well able to recognize the difference between retribution and correction and as a result may regard appropriate punishment as just and educative.

Expressing Anger is one thing, but we should generally leave the act of punishing up to karma and not create bad karma for ourselves by engaging in it. As the law of cause and effect, karma teaches people that wrong behavior is not rewarding. This may seem like punishment, but there is obviously no emotional involvement in the operation of cause and effect. If we need to punish someone because of our role in society, then we are only executors of the law of karma for that person. If, however, we punish out of Anger, in revenge, then our actions will create their own karmic impacts upon us. This not so old but famous Indian story provides an example of how to deal with this subject.

> One day a powerful trade union leader privately visited the local king. When he angrily abused the king with very impolite language, the king decided not to punish him. Instead, he gave him five gold coins and asked him not to tell anybody about what had happened between them. This freed the king from having to punish the trade leader to save his own public image. The man thought this was a great way to make money, but when he likewise insulted a very rich man, that man's bodyguards chopped off his fingers and broke his arm.

This story shows how we can add fuel to the fire of an angry person who is doing wrong things. That way he will continue his bad behavior until somebody else punishes him. This game is rather well understood by politicians.

Expressing Anger without feeling it is quite difficult. Producing harsh and loud sounds, taking an angry posture, using accusing words, and so forth all leave their mark on a person's biochemistry. For the one who wants to develop a deep inner peace, even the acting out of Anger should be avoided. Only a true saint can play any role without being emotionally affected by it.

However, if we leave the right to be angry to the "demons" alone, the world might turn into quite a horrific place. If we feel the need to act in the interest of justice and dharma, we should follow the great example given by Mahatma Gandhi. Gandhi demonstrated an Anger that was so very constructive that it can hardly be called Anger. By adhering to *satya* (truth) and *ahimsa* (non-violence), Gandhi controlled his Anger at the oppression created by the British Empire; because of it, rather than in spite of it, he helped India to gain home rule. Defending truth and justice is all right if we refrain from using violence in word, deed, or thought. Fight your enemies but do not hate or harm them. Forgive them, because they do not know what they do.

It is very helpful to realize that Anger only increases the size of any problem. Instead of just having to deal with the practical results of some injustice, getting angry means we lose our inner peace and happiness. In this way we suffer more than just through the direct result of the injustice done to us, only for the sake of righteousness. We may not be able to prevent every injustice against us, but we are the ones who can turn each injustice into a major problem, or not. We may have every right to be angry, but we also have the right not to be stupid.

Through natural justice and karma, whatever injustice is done to us, harms the doer. If we recognize this, we will also see that we have no need for Anger; then forgiveness will come easily. We should be more worried about the karmic effects of our own Anger, which represents a graver problem for us than the seeming problems of the world that prompt it. By practicing detachment from worldly possessions, from the fears and desires of the ego, from the fruits of our actions, Anger goes because expectation goes. Accept, do not expect.

While people may do bad things quite consciously, it does not mean that they are truly to blame. Deep inside, they do not want to do these things. They just lack sufficient conscious understanding and control to behave properly. Anger is always an injustice, because people always misbehave out of delusion. The one who truly understands this can forgive anybody anything and does not expect anything from anybody.

If we feel Anger but do not want it, then there are many ways to get rid of it. Indian mythology tells the story of the goddess Durga killing the demon of Anger called Mahisha. Mahisha is shown as a demon with the head of a water buffalo, because this animal can be extremely dangerous when angered, like its relatives used in the sports of bull rid-ing in the United States and bullfighting in Spain. The water buffalo's reputation of hunting down anyone that wounds it makes it feared by hunters. For the purpose of killing Mahisha, Durga was created from the combined energy of all of the gods and was provided with their weapons: The trident and other weapons from Shiva; the lotus, chakra, and other weapons from Vishnu; and so on. This symbolizes our ability to kill the demon of Anger inside of us with the help of our good and divine energies, such as forgiveness, acceptance, Calmness, Joy, and so on.

Any other Rasa can stop Anger if it is strong enough. Calmness is the opposite Rasa so if you do not want to feel Anger, you should practice prayer, meditation, and breathing exercises. Stop the breath and the Anger will stop. Or breathe slowly and deeply, in through the nose, out through the mouth.

You may also try to switch to one of the other enemy Rasas of Anger. See the humor of the situation and of your expectations. Love the enemy and understand why he or she behaves wrongly. We are all children and we all make errors that can be forgiven. Artists may express Anger in the most beautiful way and get satisfaction from it. Or we may concentrate on the Wonder of this universe and experience the relative insignificance of our problems.

Be on the watch for Anger's friendly Rasa: Fear. We must overcome the Fears that make us angry through feeling helpless.

By itself, Anger will not stay for a very long time because of the natural changes in body chemistry. So if we do not feed Anger with our thoughts, it will go all by itself.

While changing our mental attitude, we may also remove the biochemical basis for Anger. This consists of consciously cooling down the fire of Anger:

❖ Slowly drinking several glasses of cool water (not icy cold) is a sure way to get rid of Anger. Soft drinks, with a lot of sugar, acids, and often caffeine will not do. They will only increase the excitement.

❖ Drinking water that has been stored in a silver cup, accumulating lunar energy for a day and night or more, is the very best. Silver cups can be purchased in India for around ten U.S. dollars and make a priceless souvenir for anybody visiting India. As an alternative, sun-baked or unglazed clay cups may also be used.

❖ Not taking any sweet or fat and especially fasting for some time is a sure way to deny combustibles to the fire of Anger. Since the feeling of hunger may increase irritability, any food fasting should be combined with exercising Calmness.

❖ Taking a little sweet may increase kapha and reduce pitta, but only a small amount should be taken and allowed to slowly melt in the mouth, just to give the direct effect of the taste.

❖ Avoid pungent, salty, sour, and astringent tastes in general.

❖ Avoid alcohol, because it is the best combustible available, heating and drying the body.

❖ Chewing red or green cardamom will turn the acid biochemistry to alkaline and thus reduce Anger.

❖ Yogurt and lemons are very good also. Lemons are sour but are cooling, unlike most other sour foods.

❖ Wearing pearls or taking pearl powder for more than one lunar cycle is a good way to get rid of persistent Anger.*

We must, however, take care not to cool down the body too much because it may trigger a response that heats up the body, such as happens after taking a really cold shower.

It is also possible to use similar ways to reduce Anger in others, if they allow it. Anger is never ready to give up; it requires a response. If it is ignored, then it becomes stronger and might become self-destructive to the person holding it. Calm people who are respected by the angry person can try to talk him or her out of it. Really good Humor may sometimes burn the fire of Anger through laughter. For example, a woman once threatened her angry husband to commit suicide by eating sugar if he would not stop being angry. The husband could not stop himself

---

*See Harish Johari, *The Healing Power of Gemstones* (Rochester, Vt.: Destiny Books, 1996).

from laughing at the idea and his Anger disappeared. Showering Love over an angry person may satisfy the ego so that it becomes willing to let the Anger go. Doing something absolutely unexpected may cause the ego of the angry person to become numb in Wonder. The woman threatening to eat sugar actually used the Humor and Wonder Rasas both, because her reaction really astonished her husband.

Anger Sadhana

Anger Sadhana means to consciously set aside even good reasons for being angry. There may be valid reasons for being angry, but when we do Raudra Sadhana, all these good reasons are no longer important, just as food becomes unimportant when we do food fasting, even though we never question the natural need for food.

Practicing Anger Sadhana for some time will give you the power to control this Rasa at any occasion. Even if the need to express Anger in communication rises, it will be expressed without being felt, before it is felt.

Doing a sadhana of Anger means to promise yourself not to be angry in thought, word, or deed for a particular period. Not being angry in thought will require a lot of effort to keep your body chemistry balanced and cool. It will also require practicing Calmness in regular meditation.

If an angry thought comes anyway, you should accept it and deny it at the same time. Accepting it means that it should not be a reason for Anger, whether directed at yourself or at the original cause. To deny it means to put it out of your mind by analyzing the unfulfilled expectation that lies at the basis of it, which will dissolve it. If required, this contemplation of the source of the Anger may be followed by purification of the mind, such as through mantra chanting *(japa)*. In any case, the Anger should never be suppressed, only dissolved by truth, forgiveness, and purification. As long as angry thoughts keep festering inside, that job is not done.

Raudra Sadhana can be a kind of yoga adopted for a lifetime. Whoever can give up on Anger for the rest of his or her life will gain more than control over the Anger Rasa. The siddhi or power obtained by

Raudra Sadhana is *bhukti,* the power of enjoyment. Bhukti means that we get what is ours to enjoy without effort.

A very different kind of Anger Sadhana can be done in which one always remains angry. This is a demonic form of sadhana, of which the great demon Ravana makes an outstanding example. Even when Ravana was dying and Rama came in front of him, Ravana could not let his Anger go. Some people practice this sadhana without being aware of it. When maintained consciously, it can also bring a lot of power, though it is not advisable.

Rudra: The Deity of Anger

The deity of the Anger Rasa is Rudra, a wrathful aspect of Shiva. The name Rudra directly relates to the harsh sounds produced in Anger.

By pleasing Rudra as Shiva, problems with the Anger Rasa may be reduced. Pleasing Shiva means to regularly meditate, to give Love and care to all existing beings without discrimination, to work out practical solutions for the problems of humanity, to maintain a strict discipline, to reduce ignorance and remain alert.

Following is the main story about the birth of Rudra:

Once upon a time, Brahma and Vishnu sat together. When Shiva joined them in disguise, Brahma failed to recognize him and angrily insulted him. Shiva at first wanted to burn Brahma with the fire of his third eye, but when Brahma asked forgiveness, Shiva accepted the mistake made by Brahma. However, Brahma did not trust that Shiva had really forgiven him and asked for proof: He wanted Shiva to take birth as his own son. Shiva accepted. For a very long time however, nothing happened. Brahma started doubting if Shiva would keep his promise. For 5000 years, he prayed to Shiva but still nothing happened. Brahma could no longer bear it, became very angry, and committed suicide. As soon as Brahma had done this, Shiva came out of his mouth as Rudra, an angry child crying pitifully. The sound of his crying brought Brahma back from death.

Brahma was very happy to see Shiva finally incarnated as his son but started to worry about the child crying so much and so loudly. He said, "Daddy is all right, no more need for crying." However, Rudra answered that he was not crying for Brahma, but was crying in Anger because by taking birth, he had to enter the ignorance of the world and thus his inner peace was disturbed.

In this story, it is first shown how Shiva through his inherent Calmness could easily forgive Brahma, after first showing some Anger to make Brahma understand his error. That, however, created so much Fear in Brahma that he required proof of being forgiven. It also shows how when Brahma's expectations remained unfulfilled for 5000 years, Anger came and, due to the lack of response, turned into a self-destructive act. In Rudra's angry crying we see that even a god's Calmness can go when it is clouded by ignorance, creating Anger as the opposite Rasa.

RAUDRA RASA SUMMARY

Basic Rasa	Anger
Sub-Rasas	Stress, Irritability, Violence
Dominant Element	Fire
Dominant Dosha	Pitta
Dominant Guna	Rajas
Dominant Kosha	Ego (Vijnanamaya Kosha)
Friendly Rasas	Fear
Enemy Rasas	Joy, Love, Wonder
Neutral Rasas	Calmness, Courage, Sadness, Disgust
Rasa Produced	Sadness
Key for Mastering	Resist injustice if needed, but without violence or expectation
Siddhi	Bhukti (enjoyment)
Deity	Rudra

10

Veerya: Courage

*The greatest courage is to let go of pride
and admit to our mistakes.*

The Basis of Courage

Veerya or Courage is the Rasa of fearlessness, self-assurance, determination, heroism, valor, concentration, and perfect control of body and mind. When this mood is present, the ego is firmly in charge, directing body, mind, and intellect without error or hesitation. Pure Veerya is fearlessness in every sense of the word.

In ancient India, the warriors and kings who fought in accordance with the rules of dharma were known for their Veerya. The rules of war were firmly established and it was regarded as highly dishonorable and cowardly to break them. For example, fighting could only happen by day, in one to one combat, with like weaponry. This is one of the main subjects of the Mahabharata epic, in which wars were won by treachery for the first time. In Rajasthan the reputation for Courage extended to the women too, who would all commit suicide by jumping into a fire together if the odds of a battle turned against their side. Then the warriors would not have to worry about them and could fully concentrate on defending the country.

Such honorable views of war can also be found in other ancient cultures, such as in the story of the eighteenth century African king Chaka Zulu who gained power by breaking the previous code that forbade the killing of one's enemies, the Bushido codes of honor of the Japanese samurai, or the ancient saga of King Arthur and the Knights of the Round Table.

When cannon and other weapons that kill from afar started to play a role in warfare, soldiers clinging to ancient codes of honor had no choice but to march forward under fire, drummers up front, as if nothing were happening, reduced to flesh for cannon to rip apart. In modern times, war became a slaughterhouse without honor, fought with treachery, propaganda, ethnic cleansing, and powerful weapons of mass destruction that create useless grief and terror.

Still today, the Veerya Rasa lives in many people who are modern-day heroes, who serve as great examples to others and young people in particular. Some may practice the martial arts with full honor, such as the Aikido fighters that practice self-defense while maintaining the strict discipline that the attacker cannot be hurt on purpose, only deflected or restrained. Other heroes may offer their lives every day to save others, such as fire fighters or doctors that work in war and disaster zones. As sports competitions were created to substitute for war in the contests between regions and nations, so sportsmen and women replaced the warriors of old, creating admiration and awe in the spectators for their bravery, skill, and perseverance.

The list of people involved with this Rasa is endless, because Courage aids everybody when challenges need to be faced in life. This mood is very useful when we have to do something that we have never done before. Having a strong body is not a requirement for Veerya, because this Rasa can come to anybody. Essentially the Veerya Rasa relates to inner strength. In doing sadhana, Veerya is essential. Some spiritual disciplines especially require a lot of Courage, like standing on one leg or sitting in ice-cold water for a very long period.

Veerya people are very popular and that is one of the reasons why young people aspire to become heroes. Their developing egos enjoy the boost: They like showing how strong and brave they are, have many fantasies on the subject, and like to read books or watch movies that feature heroes with whom they can identify.

Sub-Rasas of Courage

There is only a thin line between Courage and pride or arrogance. When a courageous person becomes popular because of his strength and heroic deeds, the risk is high that his ego identifies with them. Pride causes a large number of problems, from the overestimation of one's abilities to war. For real Veerya, the ego must be in control and controlled at the same time.

In Bhakti Yoga, the yoga of devotion, everything that one achieves comes from God and is a part of God. This faith not only strengthens Courage, but also keeps pride at bay, creating an attitude of humility.

Courage in the Body

Veerya is dominated by the water element and rajasic in nature. Bodily strength requires water; thus kapha people are the most likely to develop Courage. Generally speaking, people with high body mass do not easily become afraid.

When the body feels less strong, as in illness, Fear and worries easily come. In addition, when the blood sugar level is low, inner strength may disappear. This is true for everyone and can particularly be seen in warriors who need to maintain bodily energy to preserve their power of determination: Hungry soldiers easily make a run for it.

Many information molecules are involved in Veerya, such as acetylcholine, adrenalin, and dopamine.

Relationship to Other Rasas

Anger is the only Rasa that is friendly to Courage, because it may strengthen it. However, the Anger must be well controlled, because Veerya needs the intellect and Anger has a tendency to overrule its advice. The tennis player John McEnroe is quite a famous expert in this matter, able to use his Anger to bring out his best shots, but sometimes also missing because of it.

Fear is an enemy Rasa to Veerya and, in fact, is its opposite. Nevertheless, when a fearful person is cornered, Courage may arise through need. Even though great Courage may be produced in defense of one's loved ones, Love is generally regarded as an enemy Rasa because it is distracting. Heroes need to defend the greater goals, not just their loved ones. Real Calmness is an enemy Rasa to Courage, because it dissolves the ego, which is essential for Veerya. While some Calmness is needed to stay in control of the body, mind, ego, and intellect, when a Veerya person encounters real Shanta, the interest in fighting for a cause disappears. Numerous stories talk of great warriors who at some point lose interest in the game of war and become hermits.

Courage most often leads to Wonder, mostly in others but also in oneself.

Mastering Courage

To become a real Veerya person requires a lot of patience and training. Whether it regards real fighting, any other physical capability, or the mental power and balance needed in any endeavor, the required neural patterns need to be developed step by step until they are real brain highways that can be taken without effort. The following story of the monkey god Hanuman is the perfect illustration of how a Veerya person requires intellect as well as physical power:

> When Hanuman flew over the ocean to the isle of Lanka in search of the abducted Sita, the gods wanted to test him. So Sursa, the goddess of snakes, blocked his path and threatened to eat him. Hanuman tried to talk her out of it and even offered to come back after fulfilling his duty in Lanka. But Sursa would not hear of it. She had received the boon that whoever came before her must pass through her mouth. But when she tried to eat him, Hanuman gradually

became bigger so that she had to open her mouth wider and wider. Suddenly Hanuman became as small as a mosquito, flew into her mouth, and back out through her ear. The boon had been fulfilled and Hanuman could continue his journey.

Along with Courage, we need to have the intelligence to become small when necessary and use our powers in a clever way.

When Courage becomes pride, it becomes destructive and self-destructive. Competition is a main aspect of the Veerya Rasa and it is very useful to test and improve our abilities. But if we take losing or winning too personally it becomes a problem. Competition requires a sportsman's spirit. If we win by unfair means, then the victory has not really been earned in the right way and its fruits will never taste as good.

Ravana is a good example of how too much ego can destroy the power of a Veerya person. Ravana had obtained the boon that he could not be killed by a god or a demon, so he became very proud, forgetting that he *could* be killed by a human. He ruled all of creation and abducted Sita by tricking Ram. That event destroyed his popularity among his own demon population and caused his downfall in the end.

Talking about whatever strength we have developed will destroy it. In these days of competition, commercialization, and promotion, it is difficult to deal with this fact. Expression of our abilities creates expectations in others; that destroys the Rasa by creating the Fear that we may not be able to live up to those expectations. Dealing with success and admiration is very hard and this problem has caused the downfall of many popular sportsmen, artists, and rulers. This aspect of Veerya is also beautifully demonstrated in a story about young Hanuman:

As a young god with extraordinary powers, Hanuman often abused them. He especially liked teasing the saints in the forest, by placing their temples in another location, drinking the water that they were offering, dousing their sacrificial fires, blowing them away with his powerful breath, and so on. Finally all the gods prayed to Brahma to find a solution. A curse was created by the saints to protect the world from the mischief of young Hanuman: They prevented him from knowing (and thus using) his own powers until Jambavant, king of the bears, reminded the grown-up Hanuman that he had extraordinary abilities.

This story teaches that whatever powers we have, we should try to forget about them and only remember them when they are needed for the sake of others and when asked to use them. We should always avoid unnecessary publicity, even if through our deeds or qualities we naturally become the center of attention.

The Courage Rasa may also bring a desire for freedom or independence, which is an illusion. Everybody and everything in this universe is interdependent. We all depend on each other; even if we feel totally self-sufficient, we still depend on the air that we breathe or on the sun to give us warmth and light. Even winning a million dollars in a lottery will make us dependent for friendship on those few people whom we can trust enough to be real friends and not just interested in our money. Dependence only becomes a problem when we have insufficient willpower to do our duties and stick to our basic needs. Then we become dependent on others who are not depending on us. A true feeling of independence and freedom only comes with self-control, when we are ready to face any challenge as required, when we know that we are valuable people upon whom other people naturally come to depend, so that we in turn may depend on them.

Courage requires a perfect balance between ego and intellect in order not to overestimate our own abilities. Veerya people like to accept all challenges but not all challenges are to be accepted. However powerful a person is, one day some task will be impossible to undertake or somebody will arise who is even more powerful. We should be prepared for this by realizing that our powers are not really ours. Again Hanuman is a perfect example. After giving Sita Rama's ring and bringing her hairclip *(chudamani)* back to Rama, he refused to accept any honor for that deed, claiming that it was first the ring and then the hairclip that gave him the power to do as he did. There is a saying that real power only stays if used in selfless service. We should be grateful to have our abilities, but should not identify with them, nor regard them as something very important.

Courage Sadhana

Maintaining any kind of discipline is Veerya Sadhana. Living according to one's dharma or duty is also Veerya Sadhana. On a basic level, it means living as perfectly as one knows how (see also chapter 18). Taken to the extreme, following dharma may be the highest Veerya Sadhana. It requires great Courage as well as great humility.

Veerya Sadhana can also mean undertaking a particularly difficult but feasible challenge in pure and selfless service. In a sadhana of selfless service or Karuna Sadhana (see chapter 11), there is no particular challenge. Only helping is necessary, whether the task is easy or difficult. In Veerya Sadhana, the exercise is to undertake a really difficult challenge for the sake of others or for spiritual growth, without any doubt and without any personal gain or feelings of pride. In pure Veerya Sadhana, no one else should even know about the deed, which is often the hardest part of it.

The siddhi obtained by Veerya Sadhana is *ishatattva,* the power to become a lord *(ish),* to be able to rule others by virtue of being free of personal objectives that go beyond basic needs.

Indra: The Deity of Courage

Indra, the king of the heavens, is the lord of the Veerya Rasa. Indra used his *vajra* (a weapon made from the spine of a rishi or seer) to destroy the great demon Vrita that represents the *vrittis,* the basic mental modifications or mental states of the mind. To control these vrittis is the task of yoga. The five sense organs and the five work organs are the ten *indriyas.* One who controls them becomes Indra. One who is a slave of them becomes Ravana Dashanana, the ten-headed demon. Controlling the mind is necessary in Veerya and requires a lot of Courage because the mind is very powerful and tricky. Indra is also famous for having complete control over prana (the life force), the clouds that represent our emotions, thunder, and lightening, and the energy created by friction. Indra also grants fearlessness.

In many stories about Indra, Courage turns into competition and pride. In one story, Indra became furious on hearing that Krishna advised people to worship the earth, the trees, and the mountains, instead of him. Indra sent a big storm to punish the people, but Krishna picked up the hill of Goverdhana on one finger and used it as an umbrella to give them all shelter. Humbled, Indra then begged forgiveness from Krishna.

As Indra represents the ego, he is very afraid of losing his kingdom. This is symbolized by many stories in which a rishi is undergoing strong austerities, and Indra fears that as a result he will become too powerful and a threat. Therefore, he tries his best to disturb that rishi by sending *apsaras* (dancing maidens) and *gandharvas* (singing men), hoping to break the concentration of Veerya Rasa by creating the Shringara Rasa.

VEERYA RASA SUMMARY

Basic Rasa	Courage
Sub-Rasas	Pride, Determination, Concentration
Dominant Element	Water
Dominant Dosha	Kapha
Dominant Guna	Rajas
Dominant Kosha	Ego (Vijnanamaya Kosha)
Friendly Rasas	Anger
Enemy Rasas	Fear, Love, Calmness
Neutral Rasas	Sadness, Disgust, Joy, Wonder
Rasa Produced	Wonder
Key for Mastering	Develop power and balance step by step and serve with humble confidence
Siddhi	Ishatattva (power to rule)
Deity	Indra

11
Karuna: Sadness

*True Compassion aims
at bringing enlightenment.*

The Basis of Sadness

Only that which is never changing is true and, in maya, everything is continuously changing. In maya, nothing lasts forever; that is the cause of suffering in those who do not see through the illusion of maya. When we feel sad for all who do not see through this illusion of suffering, for the ignorance created by maya, then we experience the highest form of Karuna, which is Compassion. Maya is the cause of Compassion for a wise person and the realization of maya is *jnana* (gyana) or real knowledge.

While the highest Karuna is Compassion, the original Sanskrit word *karuna* means "Sadness;" this more popular meaning finds expression in many kinds of art, literature, and theatre in India. The personal drama of Karna, a character of the Mahabharata epic, is a good example. Karna is the illegitimate son of Kunti and Surya, the sun god. While he was still a baby, his shamed mother put him afloat in a basket on the waters of Ganga. When he was killed during the famous battle of Kurukshetra, he had no sons to take care of his funeral rites, because all of them had been killed there as well.

Personal bad luck or something disastrous happening to one's loved ones are the most common causes for Sadness. A better understanding of the illusionary nature of existence may also create more self-centered Sadness, as in feelings that relationships with family and friends are really an illusion. Sadness is a feeling that comes when we have to let go of attachments. This pain is difficult to rationalize out of existence. When someone close dies, every culture has developed funeral rites that help us to express this feeling, so that through the expression it may also exhaust itself. In India, it is common for relatives to respect one year of mourning following a funeral, after which everybody is expected to get over the pain and get on with life.

In pity, another form of Karuna, the suffering of others is regarded as real and separate from one's own problems, even though the feeling may be stronger the more one recognizes the problem from one's own experience. The solutions thought of through pity may be well intended and offered in selfless service, but are always in vain. The only solution to suffering is true knowledge. As such, pity is a kind of suffering in sympathy, felt by a kind-hearted person, but it is still based on discrimination. For God, everything is the same and equally worthy of kindness, which is why Hindus call God "Karuna *nishan*," full of Compassion.

Compassion is a Sadness that is not self-centered. One might say that while Sadness is an ingredient of Compassion, true Compassion goes beyond Sadness to an unending kindness that doesn't taste like Sadness at all, in which the Sadness of Sadness evaporates in Love and truth.

True Compassion involves the recognition that the suffering of others (as well as their joy) is also our own. Nobody has any problem that is not related to ignorance and ignorance is the fate of all who are not enlightened. If we can feel sorry for others without feeling any better than them, we may experience the highest Karuna.

True Compassion is without discrimination and can be felt for humans as well as for animals, plants, or enemies. It makes us a kind person, extending loving kindness to every being we meet. This depth of Compassion is beautifully expressed in the story of the saint that lifted a scorpion out of the water to carry it to safety, even though it was stinging him. Both the saint and the scorpion were doing nothing but following their dharma.

Buddha did not feel pity for the suffering of others but for the ignorance that causes suffering and that is why he set himself on the path of self-realization. When becoming enlightened, the one who vows to continue to reincarnate until all beings are enlightened as well is called a Bodhisattva. The Dalai Lama is a good example of this Karuna discipline.

In Compassion, mind, ego, and intellect are active. The intellect and mind can help in analyzing both the problem and the solution. The ego has to accept a relationship in order to feel Compassion for the one who suffers. To feel Compassion for a drowning scorpion, one has to feel a kinship to it, as a saint will feel toward everything that exists.

Real Compassion is a divine quality that makes a person a real human being. This Karuna polishes our consciousness of the Divine, making it stand out more clearly and beautifully. It is the cause of many spiritual thoughts and ideas and promotes religion very well. The Christian cross is a powerful symbol of Karuna, of suffering out of Compassion for others.

Sub-Rasas of Sadness

When we feel pity for ourselves, then everything becomes sad, nothing gives joy, and we feel detached from everything. As long as we do not seek to blame anyone or our self for our misfortune, it remains just Sadness. When blame becomes the subject, then Sadness turns into Anger or Disgust. When God or life is blamed, faith is lost and the combination of Sadness, Anger, and Disgust may cause depression for a very long period.

In Bhakti Yoga, a kind of Sadness exists that is actually a part of Shringara (Vipralambha Shringara): The feeling of Sadness that comes when we feel separated from God (see chapter 5). That Sadness can be a powerful motivating force, which causes the bhakta to increase his or her efforts to reach God, the seventh chakra, and cosmic consciousness.

Sadness in the Body

Karuna is rajasic and ruled by the water element, which becomes visible when it causes tears to flow. Tears cried in self-pity are sour and harmful to the eyes. It is good that they leave the body, but the eyes should be rinsed afterward. Tears cried out of Compassion for others (or out of happiness) are not sour.

Tears more easily come to women because they are more dominated by the water element. Likewise, kapha people more easily experience the various forms of Karuna than others. Fenugreek leaves (methi), saffron, and pumpkin are great foods that can bring back joy through body chemistry.

The Moon influences the water element so it also influences our moods. Moods related to Sadness are more dominant in the descending Moon cycle. Moods that are connected with excitement and joy mostly come in the ascending cycle. At full Moon, the emotions are at a peak.

As for neurotransmitters, Sadness is mostly expressed by the absence of serotonin, dopamine, and phenylethylamine.

Relationship to Other Rasas

Hasya is an enemy Rasa of Karuna. Karuna leads to *vairagya* or non-attachment. When we experience something Sad, we feel detached from everything that normally would bring us Joy. Humor can show a sad person the trap in which he or she is caught and provide some relief. In order to achieve that goal, the joke must be of good taste, appropriate to the situation.

Likewise, Shringara is an enemy Rasa of Sadness. Embracing a sad person with Love can work miracles, as can surrounding him or her with the Beauty of nature or art. The confrontation with Shringara may bring out some tears, but that is a natural step toward recovery.

Calmness is the only friendly Rasa to Karuna, because detachment is part of both. In very severe personal Sadness, a person may become so shocked that some sort of Calmness comes as well. People who have just faced some personal disaster often outwardly look very calm because they are numbed by it.

Wonder, Courage, Anger, Fear, and Disgust are all neutral to Karuna. While true Compassion may lead to Calmness, Sadness is quite endless and most often only leads to more Sadness if not consciously changed.

Mastering Sadness

Mastering Karuna means to convert our more self-centered Sadness into genuine Compassion for our ignorance and the ignorance of others.

While real Compassion is a very saintly Rasa, a saint is not required to feel it. Especially to the tantric, everything that exists is the mother goddess, Ma or Devi. Thus for the tantric, maya ceases to be a source of Karuna and becomes the divine play called leela instead. Changing or not changing, in whatever name or form, in light or darkness, everything remains appropriate, divine, and agreeable.

As a saint is detached from self-centered desires, giving is easy. When somebody is in need or pain, help can be offered. When those needs are less pressing, truth can be offered through the very same kindness. The ability to freely give makes one saintly and sets a great example of selflessness. However, the true saint will not forget that the feeling of Compassion is just another illusion and not in itself desirable for one who sees through the illusion of maya. He will always remember that true suffering is caused by ignorance and that true help consists of bringing enlightenment. True Compassion then becomes a communication of truth in unending kindness.

Most people, however, are so absorbed by their own problems that they cannot sympathize with the problems of others. And if they do, they often do not recognize that the problems of others are not different from their own. Exercising true Compassion may help them to remove their more self-centered Sadness or pity. Thus Compassion is taught by Buddhism and Christianity; Krishna also teaches Arjuna that the first qualification for a religious person is Compassion for every being in the universe. Compassion is a major stepping-stone toward spirituality.

To directly counter any Sadness, we must first understand that Sadness may come but goes just as well. In children especially, Sadness is short-lived. The minute a problem is solved, the Sadness goes because Joy is the natural state of a child. And even if a problem cannot be solved, Sadness is easily forgotten once the attention is focused elsewhere. Bliss is our true nature; Sadness is not.

In adolescents, periods of Sadness may come when one feels neglected and tries to produce pity in others. This is also related to the desire to be loved by somebody special and to be successful. If during or shortly after adolescence a partner and success are not found, then a person may become really sad. Loneliness in general is a main cause of Sadness. Only wisdom can help here: The understanding that every problem is nothing less than an opportunity for spiritual growth.

When we get older, a Sadness may come because of waning strength and Beauty, of achievements becoming meaningless. It is then called "midlife crisis." If we accept whatever goes and find meaning in all that is still left, then there is no problem. When we understand ourselves as being truth, eternal, with no beginning and no end, with this body being just a passing phase, then that Sadness will never come. It is because we think that we are limited to this body and this life that it comes.

The same goes for the Sadness that may come when nearing death. If we believe that the end is near, then obviously Sadness will come. If we believe in eternity, then we can still enjoy everything around as a beautiful life in progress. We might for example devote our life to planting new seeds that will grow into trees and bring fruits to the coming generations. In any case, the Sadness is nothing but an error in perception.

Concentration on the enemy Rasas Love and Joy is also a very powerful way to remove Sadness. Seeing the Humor of a situation and seeking out the Joys and loved ones that still remain, will take us a long way.

Sadness Sadhana

Although some people may be sad about themselves all of their lives, that is not Karuna Sadhana. Karuna Sadhana means to deny self-centered Sadness and embrace true Compassion by being always caring and kind. While this kindness will be mostly extended to those we meet at any moment, it must be universal and undiscriminating. It is pure Karma Yoga, the dedication of one's life to the needs of the universe, without pursuing any personal gain, name, or fame. It goes beyond dedicating one's life to a cause—the entire universe is embraced with Compassion.

One who performs such Karuna Sadhana without ego achieves the siddhi called *mahima* or mightiness, the power to be as big as one desires. Then one can even be nailed on a cross and still teach the entire world a lesson of Compassion.

Varuna: The Deity of Sadness

The deity of Karuna is Varuna, the lord of water. Water is life *(jivan)* and life flows like water. Water is also the essence of all Rasas and in Karuna it comes out as tears.

Varuna causes rains to fall and rivers to flow and continuously evaluates the actions of human beings. He is the keeper of the laws of dharma, because following one's dharma means to cause minimal Sadness in others as in oneself. He is the guardian of the sea of heaven and overlord of the terrestrial seas. His palace is situated on the submerged mountain Pushpagiri. The souls of the drowned ones go to him, attended by nagas or snakes. Among the elder Vedic deities, Varuna is generally seen by historians as the first morally righteous, kind, and benevolent god, ready to forgive the transgressions of the devotee.

Obviously, Buddha himself might be a likely candidate for being a Karuna lord, because Compassion is at the very basis of Buddhist teachings.

KARUNA RASA SUMMARY

Basic Rasa	Sadness
Sub-Rasas	Compassion, Pity
Dominant Element	Water
Dominant Dosha	Kapha
Dominant Guna	Rajas
Dominant Kosha	Ego
Friendly Rasas	Calmness
Enemy Rasas	Joy, Love
Neutral Rasas	Disgust, Wonder, Anger, Fear, Courage
Rasa Produced	Sadness
Key for Mastering	Kindly embrace both truth and ignorance
Siddhi	Mahima (mightiness)
Deity	Varuna

12

Bhayanaka: Fear

When there is nothing to lose,
there is nothing to Fear.

The Basis of Fear

Bhay in Sanskrit means "fear," and Bhayanaka means "full of fear, fearful, terrified." Fear is often caused by ignorance. When something is unknown, the mind can only imagine what it can do and if the ego is not confident enough, the mind will only imagine fearful things. In the pure ignorance of a baby, there is no Fear. For Fear to come, we must be conscious of being ignorant.

When we feel confident, that same ignorance may just as well bring the excitement and curiosity of the Wonder Rasa. Fear is primarily a game of the ever-exaggerating mind, while the ego suffers from it if it identifies with it. The intellect obviously may try to help by offering explanations and solutions, but if the ego has already surrendered to Fear, it will be of no avail.

The most powerful expression of the Rasa Fear is the fear of death. While death comes only once in life, the fear of death may last a lifetime. To the dying person, a strong sense of fear usually comes when the prana starts withdrawing from the feet, which become numb as a result. When the brain also starts to fail, the fear may become a suffocating feeling.

As many desires exist, so many fears may arise. They are all fears of future failure and loss. The more responsibilities we have, the more projects we undertake, the more fearful we may become. The more we are attached to whatever we have or might obtain, the more reason for the Fear Rasa.

In society, Fear is one of the Rasas that makes people respect law and authority. There is a saying in India that every respectful man is afraid of his wife. And of course, Fear is our natural protection that keeps us away from harm.

Sub-Rasas of Fear

Worries are a minor form of Fear. Modern human beings who live in peaceful areas have little to really Fear, because we encounter very few life-threatening situations compared to more ancient people who constantly needed to be on their guard for predators and other natural dangers. On the other hand, modern humans may have a lot more possessions, projects, and relationships to worry about and some people are unable to stop worrying all the time. To worry means to live in the future and as such it takes most enjoyment out of life today.

Nervousness is another form of Fear in which there often is no clear reason for the Fear but a general state of Fear or restlessness that causes one to jump at every sound or shadow. This state is caused by too much worrying or a particular experience that caused severe anxiety. As Fear and Anger are friendly Rasas, nervousness may contain both.

Another important kind of Fear is jealousy, when we Fear the loss of someone's love. Jealousy is an explosive state of rapidly shifting between the Rasas of Love, Fear, Disgust, and Anger. It may cause a person to become quite insane and act accordingly. It is the mood that can cause murders of passion.

Fear in the Body

Fear is rajasic and dominated by the air element, which causes fearful people to tremble and shake and causes the stomach to contract. If the air element is disturbed, the mind becomes very excited and hard to control. It speeds up the heartbeat and the breathing rate. The mind is not limited to the brain but includes the entire body. In Fear, all body cells scream at us to run for our lives.

When sudden Fear is triggered by an outer cause or an inner thought, a metallic taste can be sensed in the mouth. That is the taste of akasha or ether, the element of imagination in Fear. Akasha is not directly involved in any Rasa, but because air contains akasha and as Fear creates lots of air, the taste of akasha can be experienced.

Vata dominated people worry more easily than others do and, generally speaking, women worry more easily than men, because caution is built into the body chemistry of every mother. To reduce worries and anxiety, wearing pearls and eating pearl powder is a very good medicine. Other gems may help in case of Fear, such as turquoise, which reduces the Fear of traveling, or red coral, which alleviates the Fear of thunder, lightening, and drowning.

The glucose in our blood is the main food of our brain, so if our blood sugar level is too low, the brain will not function properly and will create distress signals that may cause nervousness and anxiety. Adrenalin, dopamine, melatonin, serotonin, and noradrenalin are neurotransmitters that affect Fear.

Relationship to Other Rasas

Anger and Fear are companion Rasas that stimulate each other. Even though they cannot coexist at a single moment, we can easily move from Fear to Anger and vice-versa. Modern psychology calls this the fight-or-flight response. Fear of an unknown threat may turn into Anger when the threat becomes more defined and that Anger may again turn into Fear if met by even stronger Anger.

Wonder and Fear are related because most wondrous things cause a minimal amount of Fear; our inability to comprehend them makes us cautious.

Courage, Calmness, Joy, and Love will all remove Fear. Courage or

Fearlessness is the opposite Rasa. In Calmness, the air element becomes balanced. In Joy, the cause of Fear loses power. In Love, we feel protected by others.

Disgust and Sadness or Compassion are neutral to Fear. They neither stimulate it nor reduce it.

The Rasa most often produced following Fear is Anger, whether it happens by facing the threat or after running away from it. The coward only becomes angry at a safe distance.

Mastering Fear

Fear can be overcome by inner strength, Love, and truth. When we see only unity in diversity, there is no Fear because there is no ignorance. In truth, there is nothing to be afraid of. Deities and saints often hold one hand in the mudra (hand posture) of the Fearlessness that is only offered by truth.

By improving our inner strength, we gain more control over our body, mind, ego, and intellect. When body and mind are shut down in deep sleep, we Fear nothing. Sometimes we can eat without tasting, look without seeing, and hear without listening, because our mind is involved elsewhere. If that which causes us Fear or worry is analyzed by the intellect as nothing to be afraid of or as nothing that we can actually avoid, we should direct our mind's attention elsewhere. Holding the breath or slowing down the breath are the best ways to instantly reduce the excitement of our mind. The more we improve our control over mind, the more our self-confidence will grow.

Fear regards the future, far and near. When we look at our past and all the plans we made for it, we come to realize that our planning has really had little impact on what happened. Much more important in the determination of the course of past events have been unforeseeable, unplanned problems as well as opportunities, our karmic destiny. We must accept that for the future it will be no different. All we can do is be prepared to make the best use of every problem and opportunity that comes our way. The future will take care of itself, so let us not sacrifice today's happiness because of it.

Fear only really goes when the ego goes, because it is the ego that identifies with the body and its projects and possessions. The mind is a tricky monkey that easily jumps out of control, but the ego is responsible for allowing it to do so. Either the ego must be made so strong that we Fear nothing, or we should stop identifying with the body, projects, and possessions. When we have nothing to lose then there is nothing to Fear. The more we collect the more we can lose. To live without Fear, live on basic needs.

Real knowledge of truth brings fearlessness, while more knowledge of the world brings Fear. The fear of death is really the fear of ego for its own existence, which is an illusion. If we are not real then our ghosts cannot be real, so why would maya be afraid of maya? Meditation on the third eye makes us move beyond body consciousness and that will eventually remove all Fear.

Love and friendship can also overcome Fear. In company, we may feel more protected. The Love of a saint may remove our Fear if we believe in it. If not then a thousand saints cannot remove it. When we read scriptures or sing bhajans near a dying person, it may help them to overcome the Fear of having to leave this world.

Fear Sadhana

Fear Sadhana is rather complicated, because there is a thin line between worrying and planning ahead. That makes it very hard to evaluate whether we are still following the sadhana or not. In Fear Sadhana, we should make a clear distinction between planning and worrying.

Whatever worrying thought comes up, we must evaluate if the subject has been properly studied and appropriate action has been planned. If not then that is allowed. If a plan already exists, we must stop ourselves from going over it repeatedly because that is defined as worrying. For example, we may plan when to buy food for the evening dinner, but once that is done it is no use to worry about it any longer. We should accept that no amount of planning can ever foresee all potential obstructions.

It is also very important to make the distinction between planning and worrying because very often people do not make proper plans for dealing with a particular problem even though they worry about the problem very often. The Fear that no plan can be devised to cover the entire problem then creates a blockage in our thoughts. In Fear Sadhana, that Fear should also be overcome.

If we neglect our duty, then worrying becomes a duty. A saint will not have many duties that require planning. A householder will. When we have a problem in doing our duties, in following our dharma, it is essential that we perform Duty Sadhana (see chapter 18) before attempting any Fear Sadhana. Otherwise the Fear Sadhana may just become an excuse for acting even less responsibly.

This way, gradually, we may become so truly Fearless that even planning ahead is no longer needed because whatever happens is fine. That sadhana will give us the power of *ichcha,* the power of accomplishment, omnipotence. Whatever we want to do, we will be able to do.

Yama: The Deity of Fear

As the Fear of death is the greatest Fear, Yama, the lord of death, rules this Rasa. In Vedic belief, Yama was the first mortal to die so he is quite an expert on the matter. Yama lives in the Hindu underworld called the Patala Loka, where he guides the dead toward new life.

In the Katha Upanishad, the story of Nachiketa and Yama teaches that the Self does not die when the body dies. Through meditation and grace, the Self can be known and immortality can be achieved by breaking the cycle of birth, death, and rebirth.

BHAYANAKA RASA SUMMARY

Basic Rasa	Fear
Sub-Rasas	Worry, Nervousness, Anxiety, Jealousy
Dominant Element	Air
Dominant Dosha	Vata

BHAYANAKA RASA SUMMARY (continued)

Dominant Guna	Tamas
Dominant Kosha	Mind (Manomaya Kosha)
Friendly Rasas	Wonder, Anger
Enemy Rasas	Courage, Calmness, Joy, Love
Neutral Rasas	Disgust, Sadness
Rasa Produced	Anger
Key for Mastering	Seek company and truth while doing your duty
Siddhi	Ichcha (omnipotence)
Deity	Yama

13

Vibhatsa: Disgust

No Rasa is more demonic and useless than Disgust.

The Basis of Disgust

Vibhatsa is a feeling of Disgust or dissatisfaction with oneself and others. Vulgar, uncivilized, and perverted actions, using bad words and manners, and showing bad intentions to others are all manifestations of the Vibhatsa Rasa. Eventually, severe depression alternated with fits of craziness may be witnessed. In modern times the pressure to perform and excel is so strong that Disgust comes more easily than in times past.

Though the problem is basically mental and supported by bad body chemistry, the ego has the power to control it or to surrender to it. The ego may lose the power to control Vibhatsa if it has been deeply hurt by seeing bad intentions behind the words and deeds of others, making the person feel cheated. When the ability to judge these intentions properly is dissolved by frustration about the failure to avoid being hurt or to avoid hurting, dissatisfaction with oneself and others results. If, on the contrary, the ego has not been hurt in any major way, it can resist the pull of both body and mind that lures it into the trap of underestimating oneself.

Vibhatsa usually develops when the mind notices a word or an event that represents or brings a reminder of hurt caused by the egotism of others or unaccepted behavior of oneself. If bad body chemistry supports it, a feeling of dissatisfaction is suddenly produced, though its origin usually remains unclear to the one experiencing it. The person just suddenly feels bad. Associations with old and recent memories of one's own failures, followed by a malicious predicting of purely hypothetical failures of the future, may further strengthen the Rasa. In severe Vibhatsa, the mind spins a powerful spiral of negative thinking, shutting down the objective advice of the intellect, seeming to leave the ego with no alternative but to feel dissatisfied with everything, to cower before its responsibilities, and cut itself off.

With the mind freely wielding negative thoughts and illusions of sense- and self-gratification, Vibhatsa leads to the neglect of responsibilities, often with regard to one's health and loved ones. Strength and will are destroyed—ego becomes the king that has forsaken his country. This neglect creates deteriorating, highly tamasic body chemistry, and new failures in daily life, only further securing the chains of the trap. It also creates bad karma.

At this stage, the self-underestimating ego may frantically try to get attention from others by acting in ways that are disgusting. It then lacks sufficient contact with the intellect to realize that such attention will only be negative if one pays no attention to others' feelings of appropriateness, whether personal or cultural.

Vibhatsa forms the basis for organized as well as senseless crime. It is the most demonic Rasa and the only Rasa that really is not desirable. It may represent justice and punishment for bad body chemistry and for imbalance. It forces one to improve balance, by taking away all balance. However, there is no bottom to this pool of darkness, except where the ego decides enough is enough and starts directing the energy upward again. It is much better if the ego can decide in the first place that the road to nowhere is not a smart choice when one has become temporarily lost.

Sub-Rasas of Disgust

Depression is a complex emotional state that involves the Disgust Rasa as self-contempt and dissatisfaction, but also includes Sadness and Fear. The person that chooses depression instead of Disgust has enough sense of appropriateness left to generally avoid disgusting behavior. Nevertheless, severe dissatisfaction with oneself is still at the basis of it, even if the expression is more of Sadness, uncertainty, and inaction.

Shame is a form of Disgust, in which one recognizes one's own faults, feels dissatisfied with oneself because of it, and fearful of other people's judgment.

Disgust in the Body

Vibhatsa is a little Anger, a little fire, drowned in too much water. Just as water can find one little weakness in a roof, a small mistake may cause a person to feel Disgust for his or her entire being. Water is a great solvent, and can absorb almost anything. It can be tasteless, salty, sweet, heavenly scented, or rotten. In Disgust, it is the latter. Kapha dominated people are most easily caught by it.

Prolonged Sadness, Anger, Fear, and Disgust all relate to tamasic body chemistry. Constipation is a major cause for Disgust. The continuous spreading of toxins produced by the rotting of food in the intestines makes it impossible to develop finer feelings. Likewise, feelings of Disgust may severely disturb digestion, producing nausea and even vomiting. Disgusting smells and sights may also have these effects.

Even if somebody tries to hide feelings of Disgust, it can be easily detected because it causes the unconscious lifting of one side of the mouth, usually the left.

CRF, cholecystokin, phenylethylamine, serotonin, and noradrenalin all play a role in Disgust.

Relationship to Other Rasas

Disgust can be stimulated by the Rasas of Anger, Courage, and Wonder. A particular cause of Anger becomes just another reason to express Disgust. Feelings of Wonder at one's capacity to provoke others only increase the Courage to take it even further. When a disgusted person is confronted with wonderful deeds of others, it often just stimulates the negative self-image.

Shringara as Love and Beauty is the enemy Rasa that can be used to cure Disgust. Expressing Love and receiving Love keeps the ego satisfied with itself and others and helps to remove the attention from past suffering from the egotism of others. Creating a beautiful atmosphere brings the mind to a higher level.

The Rasa most often produced by Disgust is Fear. Other people have no idea what the crazy person may do next and will try to keep a distance. When the feeling of Disgust has subsided, the person that expressed it becomes fearful of the consequences.

Mastering Disgust

Vibhatsa is mostly avoided by frequently paying attention to Shringara. Good company may certainly help from the moment that Vibhatsa is sufficiently controlled to allow oneself to enjoy the company of others and to become enjoyable company oneself. At all times, one should keep busy, preferably in a useful way.

Friendliness and respect to others prevent the expression of bad intentions both ways. Ignoring the egotism of others, without becoming naive or easy game, offers strong protection. It makes it their problem, which it really is.

Paying attention to one's health avoids bad body chemistry. Using sufficiently hot spices helps digestion and avoids the overpowering by tamas. The air element can be easily mastered by proper food and proper circulation, so that gases do not disturb the system. The fire element can be easily mastered by proper nourishment, so that the required energy is always available. The water element is best mastered by surrender to a particular cause or discipline.

The best reaction to feelings of Disgust is to ignore them, recognizing that they lead nowhere but downward. When Vibhatsa is first detected, it can be stopped from further developing by holding the breath. Vibhatsa is a game of the mind whose restlessness may be restrained through breathing exercises. The body must be relaxed and its chemistry must become more alkaline. One should take some fruits or juices, astringent or bitter tastes, that provide the liver with help to purify the blood. Lift the mood with good music, some sightseeing, and so on.

People who follow a spiritual path may sometimes feel dissatisfied with their inability to put the theory into practice. One should accept that understanding and knowing are two different things. Achieving real knowledge not only requires effort, but also experience, time, and the grace of God. One should trust in one's divine qualities and in the method followed.

The main task in mastering Disgust is to simply stop negative identification. When we identify with bad thoughts and deeds of the past, how can we improve? When we feel doomed by destiny, we are truly lost. To fully master Disgust we should only identify with our divine nature and see our weaknesses as past errors of judgment.

When longer periods of Vibhatsa persist, confidence and will must be strengthened. Alone or with the help of others, one must develop the witnessing consciousness, deeply understanding that one may well be caught by various trips or traps, but one is neither the trip nor the trap. Trips end and traps can be avoided. One should watch the play until it becomes clear that the one who feels disgusted does not exist and holds power only if regarded as real. When we recognize our confident Self as the true reality, we can accept the necessity of training the ego and mind in order to maintain that confidence.

Strict disciplines are a great help, such as food fasting, diet fasting, sleep fasting, and speech fasting. They also purify the body chemistry and the senses. Whenever one feels dissatisfied, one should immediately start food fasting. No matter what chemical build-up is in the body, the feeling will disappear within two days of fasting.

Confidence gives us control over all Rasas, and Vibhatsa is no exception. And we should always remember that the exercise of Shringara is needed to remove the hurt from the ego. Life must be enjoyed. Overconfidence is, however, to be avoided, as new Vibhatsa can thus be created the moment one crashes into new failures, which are a natural attribute of the path of karma.

Sometimes in Disgust, people have become so discouraged, so unsure of themselves, that they really need support to slowly regain confidence.

Disgust Sadhana

As Disgust makes no sense at all, Disgust Sadhana is easy in the sense that it is a very clear sadhana to perform. Disgusting thoughts, words, or actions are simply not allowed. It may be difficult for people who are often depressed or dissatisfied to imagine, but Disgust Sadhana is really the easiest sadhana to undertake. The moment one mentally blocks any developing Vibhatsa, it stands no chance.

On the other hand, modern society is very tolerant toward disgusting expressions, such as in language (take the f-word). When doing Vibhatsa Sadhana one will need to taste every word and deed in relation to its proper quality and not simply follow society's norms, which are tainted.

The siddhi that results from doing Vibhatsa Sadhana is *prakam*, the power to assume any form, to be whatever you desire.

Mahakala: The Deity of Disgust

Mahakala is a form of Shiva. He is husband to Kali and both are destroyers of imbalance. Mahakala is the lord of time and death and is often shown in Tibetan *tankas* as the wheel of time. Time is measured in death only, because for eternal beings time has no meaning. Mahakala reminds us that nothing in maya lasts forever, Disgust included.

Mahakala is the deity of the Vibhatsa Rasa, sent to us as a purifying punishment for our mistakes, our deviations from dharma. The feeling that something is not right and we are not doing the right things forces us toward change and our rightful dharma. Therefore, Mahakala is also a symbol of natural justice.

VIBHATSA RASA SUMMARY

Basic Rasa	Disgust
Sub-Rasas	Depression, Dissatisfaction, Vulgarity
Dominant Element	Water
Dominant Dosha	Kapha
Dominant Guna	Tamas
Dominant Kosha	Mind (Manomaya Kosha)
Friendly Rasas	Wonder, Anger, Courage
Enemy Rasas	Love
Neutral Rasas	Joy, Sadness, Fear, Calmness
Rasa Produced	Fear
Key for Mastering	Ignore it and stop negative identification, while turning to purification
Siddhi	Prakam (power to assume any form)
Deity	Mahakala

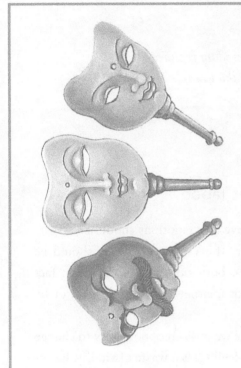

PART THREE

*Working
with
Our Rasas*

14

Mastering Emotions

True emotional freedom requires
control over the Rasas.

The Great Taboo

Many people in modern society believe that emotions should be largely ignored and suppressed, while others think that everybody should be able to freely express their emotions. Both sides in this debate in fact uphold a taboo on mastering emotions, either by ignoring them or by identifying with them too much.

When we ignore unhappy feelings we miss an opportunity to change them. Ignoring or suppressing happy feelings is a waste of vitality. Ignoring emotions simply does not work, because they come and go anyway. A baby may not know which side is up or down, but it is born with Love and Sadness, Joy and Anger. Any parent can confirm that. Living life without emotions is empty. The attitude that ignores emotions in fact originates within an emotion itself: the Fear of letting go of mental defenses, the Fear of being absorbed by an unpleasant mood, the Fear of losing a pleasant mood. Those fears can be controlled.

Emotional "freedom fighters" are reacting against the real problems caused by too much suppression of emotions. However, we should be grateful that people do not always freely express their emotions. Anger usually generates more Anger and that kind of interaction often leads to violence. And if we have the courage to look deeply inside, we must come to the conclusion that it is hard to even think about some very personal emotions. To communicate them to others in a valuable way requires a specific audience at a specific time and place.

But some peace in society is not the only reason why mastering emotions is important. In most cases, Anger, Fear, Sadness, and Disgust make no sense and Love, Joy, Wonder, Courage, or Calmness make a lot of sense. Identification with less agreeable emotions will only make them stronger. If something is displeasing, getting upset about it only makes it a lot worse. Too much identification with agreeable emotions will only make it more difficult to accept that they are time-bound and may undermine their strength. True freedom only comes when we are fully in control.

Identifying with our emotions leads to delusion because they really are not ours. In order to understand this we only need to close our eyes and try not to think any thoughts or feel any emotions. Unless we have mastered meditation, thoughts and feelings will come, even if we are trying hard to avoid them. How can they be ours if they come without our asking them to? Why do they stay even when we do not want them? Who is the one that experiences them and likes them or not? Who or what is creating them if we are not? Emotions and thoughts are only as real as we make them.

Rasa Sadhana or the "Yoga of Emotion" is not about rationalizing our emotions all the time. Rather, it is important to think and rationalize about them when reading this book, and now and then afterward as well. It is also important to practice exercising control over our emotions. The experience gained through performing such exercises or sadhana will enable us to consciously use a number of tricks that let us stay in charge for as much or as little as we like while our emotions change. After some time this will also happen through more unconscious reflexes.

Choose Sadness or Joy

One Rasa naturally leads to another. Everybody is absolutely free and able to move from any Rasa to any other Rasa. Nevertheless, some general routes are the most obvious or common:

There are only three possible end results in this scheme: Joy, Sadness, or Calmness. Love leads to Joy, as does Courage through Wonder. Disgust produces Fear most often, which further is likely to create Anger, resulting in Sadness. These routes have been explained for each Rasa in Part 2.

Most of all, this overview shows that our choices are limited: We end up in either Joy or Sadness. Or we may choose Calmness for its own sake or as an intermediate phase to move from a less desirable Rasa to a more desirable Rasa. It is up to each of us. Any rational person will choose the Rasas that ultimately bring Joy and will try to avoid those that ultimately lead to Sadness.

Calmness can be a very handy way to temporarily stop the game of Rasas and turn it in a more favorable direction. When a computer starts giving too many errors, it is time to press the "reset button" or

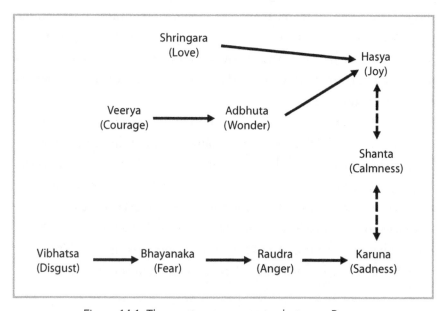

Figure 14.1 The most common routes between Rasas.

even "shut down" and "restart." Similarly, in Calmness, we choose to temporarily stop our mind and the Rasas, so that we can restart our biocomputer with a clean slate. If things are so bad that there is no more interest in Joy-full Rasas, then Calmness is always the best option and we need nobody else to create it. If Calmness stays long enough, it will either continue or, with a little help, Joy will come peeping around the corner. If Joy is not an option and it also doesn't seem the right time for Calmness, then Courage or self-confidence is the only remaining agreeable Rasa for which we do not depend on others.

Rasas of Preference

A very important step in Rasa Sadhana is to consciously choose our personal Rasa of preference. That Rasa needs to be exercised specifically, integrated within our daily life and placed at the center of our desires. Whenever the opportunity arises, we should turn to it. Whenever we feel dissatisfied, it will satisfy. Consciously satisfying the very essential desire for that Rasa will strongly reduce all other desires and create the basis for a happy and fulfilling life.

A principal attraction to specific Rasas is often formed in adolescence. This is the age when our very personal tastes are largely created, because at that age there are times when everything feels really perfect and other times when everything feels really, really bad. It is in fact the age when the Rasas are both physically and mentally at their peak, so the strongest emotions that we experience at that age determine our later preferences.

Our Rasa of preference is the Rasa that we desire the most. To find out which of the nine Rasas is a likely candidate, there are many possible approaches. However, it is most essential to ask which Rasa has given us our peak enjoyment in life. That peak may have occurred only once in our lifetime or more often. We have to analyze our memory and may need some real courage to accept the result. That peak or those peaks of enjoyment will have created a very strong desire for that Rasa. If ignored, remaining satisfied with life becomes very difficult.

For many people who are interested in spirituality, householders or not, the Calmness Rasa is an obvious choice. If one has really tasted the peace of deep meditation even once, then the desire for more is difficult to ignore. Other suitable candidates may be the moods of spiritual devotion, artistic creativity, selfless service, wonder in face of the Divine and the "not this—not that" humor that arises from the Yoga of Knowledge (Jnana Yoga), which sees the never changing in and through the ever-changing illusion of maya. For most people, spiritual or not, the main desire is to meet the love of their life, so Shringara is a very popular Rasa of preference.

Each person has one or two Rasas that are naturally dominant and for which one has the most "talent." This talent strongly depends on body chemistry and the dominant doshas:

DOMINANT DOSHAS OF THE RASAS

Kapha (Mucus) Water and Earth	Pitta (Bile) Fire and Air	Vata (Wind) Air and Akasha
Love	Joy	Calmness
Courage	Wonder	Fear
Sadness	Anger	
Disgust		

Some people are dominated by one dosha, others by two doshas, and some have all three doshas more or less in balance. In order to gain some idea of the category to which you belong, the following overview may be helpful:

SOME CHARACTERISTICS OF THE DOSHAS

	Kapha	Pitta	Vata
Type	Introvert	Centrovert (centered, balanced)	Extrovert
Sleeps	A lot	Average	Little
Talks	Less	Confidently	A lot

	Kapha	Pitta	Vata
Memory	Strong	Average	Weak
Mind	Stable	Kind or Angry	Restless
Hair	Thick	Early white	Thin, brittle
Eyes	Smooth	Reddish	Round, dry
Build	Full	Strong	Tall, thin
Health	Good	Average	Weak

It is best if an Ayurvedic doctor determines dosha dominance, because it really requires researching many more parameters. Then it becomes possible to determine more correctly which Rasas are the most suited to one's biochemistry:

❖ People who are very kapha dominated are the most emotional of all three types. It is best for them to concentrate on Love and Courage. Their ideal occupation is their home, family, art, decoration, and devotion. Karuna can be an option if they are mature enough to put it to good use in real Compassion and selfless service. Disgust and Sadness are the primary traps, which will require the most Rasa Sadhana to change. Sadhanas of Anger and Fear will be easier to manage.

❖ For people who are very pitta dominated, Joy is the best option and they should try to avoid Anger as much as possible. Wonder is not really a matter of choice, though pitta people may try to be open-minded to the miracles of the world in order to subdue their ego. They mostly need Anger Sadhana, while the Sadhanas of Sadness, Disgust, and Fear will be easier for them.

❖ For vata dominated people, practicing Calmness and controlling Fear are extremely important. An overactive mind is the main problem. As vata carries the other doshas, other options are available as well, but without some mastery of Calmness, primarily the less desirable Rasas will arise. Fear Sadhana is the biggest challenge for vata people, while Sadhanas of Anger, Disgust, and Sadness will be easier to handle.

For people who have two or three more or less equally dominating doshas, there are more options. Nevertheless, it is still important for them to identify their Rasa of preference, even though it may be for a specific period rather than for a lifetime. Only concentration on a limited subject can bring real mastery.

Our personal "talent" for particular Rasas can also be discovered through astrology and numerology. For example, the Anger Rasa relates to Mars and the number nine, according to Vedic astrology and numerology. The Love Rasa relates to Venus and the number six. The Fear Rasa often causes problems in people who are strongly influenced by the Moon or the number two. The Disgust Rasa often creates problems for people with the number eight or a badly afflicted Saturn. Calculation of the numbers mentioned can be done according to the Vedic numerology book of Harish Johari.*

For everyone, mastering all Rasas is needed for a successful life. To dwell in one or two Rasas most of the time, we need to be able to handle the others when they are needed or manifest themselves naturally. Therefore, we should choose our Rasa of preference well, and place it at the center of our attention, but not become too attached to it.

---

*Harish Johari, *Numerology, with Tantra, Ayurveda, and Astrology* (Rochester, Vt.: Destiny Books, 1990).

15

Rasa Sadhana

Sincere sadhana allows anybody to become a Rasa master.

Reprogramming the Brain

Rasa Sadhana is an ancient tantric method of changing neural and bio-chemical patterns, with which we take up the challenge of altering our emotional patterns all the way to the level of the structure of our brain. While various parts of the brain have various functions, no function of the brain can be completely limited to one area; thinking and emotional processes require communication between many parts of the brain. The quality of this communication partly depends on the links that are present between those parts. Some parts of the brain are strongly linked in almost everybody, while some people create more unique links between parts of the brain or have a deficiency in links compared to others. In women, for example, connections between the left and right hemispheres of the brain are more developed than in men, on average.

Both overdeveloped links and undeveloped links can interfere with our emotional health. In fact, many of the most persistent neural patterns are emotional in nature. The part of the limbic brain called the amygdala is a major cause for emotional distress. A strong connection exists between the eyes and the amygdala, allowing the amygdala to create a response to visual threats even before the forebrain has the time to process the incoming information. It may save our life, but it may also keep us from developing balanced, rational reactions to certain stimuli.

While the techniques of Rasa Sadhana are simple to understand, we still need time and practice to overcome our tendencies to become stuck in certain thought patterns and typical emotional responses. This is especially true when we have been stuck for a long period of time. This is very clear in people who have experienced some trauma or other and as a result react compulsively to certain stimuli. Less traumatic but prolonged unpleasant experiences may also cause people to become caught in certain patterns of behavior.

Despite the strength of such patterns, Rasa Sadhana enables us to activate our capacity to change them. It has been demonstrated that, for example, with enough time and effort even heroin addicts have been able to restore their natural ability to produce endorphins.

Setting Objectives

Depending on your biochemistry, personal preferences, and temporary problems or opportunities, you may choose which Rasa to exercise. It is generally not advisable to try to master two Rasas at the same time. It is better to concentrate on one Rasa until you are satisfied with the result, then start on another one, while maintaining the first sadhana, or not.

Attempting to master a less agreeable Rasa such as Anger, Fear, Sadness, or Disgust by mastering the opposite agreeable Rasa is not a very good method. In general it is advisable to first fast *from* the less agreeable Rasas and then increase Rasa mastery by working with the agreeable Rasas. Fasting *on* one of the agreeable Rasas is more difficult because it is not always possible or acceptable to society for a person to remain in one particular Rasa, such as when somebody expresses nothing but Wonder, no matter what happens. It is less likely for people to expect a person to remain in one of the disagreeable Rasas, so society is more naturally supportive of sadhanas that seek to master them.

Among the less agreeable Rasas, Disgust is usually the best one to tackle first, because it is the only Rasa that never makes sense and has the worst effect on our emotional well-being and on our biochemistry. When one completely avoids being dissatisfied with oneself and with one's destiny or karma, life becomes a lot more enjoyable. Disgust usually generates Fear, so it is difficult to master Fear without mastering Disgust. After mastering Disgust, the sadhana of Anger is a logical choice, followed by sadhanas of Sadness and Fear. Nevertheless, those choices are quite personal. Rasa Sadhana should be undertaken for any Rasa that causes problems.

Once we achieve control over our less desirable emotions, they will no longer disturb our natural tendencies toward more agreeable feelings. Then Love, Joy, Wonder, Calmness, Courage, and Compassion will arise very naturally. When we are no longer annoyed by the disagreeable Rasas, we automatically perform some kind of sadhana that includes all agreeable Rasas. While that is the most agreeable approach to life itself, it still remains important to work on each of them individually.

Instead of fasting from a particular type of emotion that we need to avoid, we then start fasting on a specific emotion that we want to enhance. Even if the sadhana lasts only for an hour, it teaches us how to keep that Rasa steady and pure. A person who has truly mastered the agreeable emotions can effortlessly shift to them according to need. While positive thinking can be beneficial, it is largely an intellectual game that happens on the surface of the mind and thus has limited impact. With the mastery gained by Rasa Sadhana on the agreeable Rasas, however, positive feelings radiate from all levels of our being, changing the entire environment around us, up to the very stuff this universe is made of: to the point where even molecules and atoms start vibrating on the same level and miracles can happen.

A prolonged Sadhana of Calmness is very difficult for a householder, except perhaps on vacation. Nevertheless, regularly performing Calmness exercises is essential for the practice of any Rasa Sadhana. Such exercises need only take from a quarter of an hour to an hour or more.

Calmness is ever an option if we wish to counter any Rasa. No Rasa can stay when Calmness starts to dominate, because Calmness is ni-rasa, without Rasa.

For other agreeable Rasas, the choice is really very personal, as explained in chapter 14.

Setting the Rules

It is important to clearly establish the rules of a particular sadhana, because otherwise the sadhana can be very destructive to one's self-confidence.

It is best to avoid talking about sadhana to others, as sadhana requires Courage and talking about one's Courage destroys self-confidence (see chapter 10). In some cases, not talking about the sadhana can be a part of the rules, because if others know about it, it might become too easy or too difficult to maintain the rules. In Anger Sadhana for example, talking about it to others might cause them to try to test you or, on the other hand, to become particularly soft on you.

The main rule to set is the duration of the sadhana. It is advisable to keep it short in the beginning and gradually increase the duration. It should be a challenge that you feel able to meet. Rasa Sadhana is often more difficult than expected because emotions tend to come and go as they please and it is important not to fail. If you finish with a sadhana of one day, you may start the next one for another day or a week, preferably leaving one "normal" day in between. A sadhana of twenty-eight days is a minimum to achieve some real mastery of a Rasa. It is best to start a long-term sadhana in the ascending Moon cycle.

Other rules relate to the particular Rasa, as explained in Part 2 of this book. Nevertheless, you are free to be creative about it and use any occasion to exercise a Rasa. Suppose a Westerner arrives in New Delhi with one day left before needing to catch a plane home. A great Anger and Fear Sadhana would be to make the scary one-hour journey from the center of the city to the airport without paying the taxi driver one rupee more than Indian people would, without getting angry or worried in the process. This is just an exercise—generally it is quite all right to pay a little more than Indian people would.

Another example is to take a vow never to become angry with a particular person, one who is generally quite good at making you angry. Or, if you are having money problems, you can vow to always open any new bills immediately on their arrival. Yet another would be to find a new miracle of life to wonder about every day, immediately after waking.

It is most important to avoid bending the rules while the sadhana is going on. However, if you have made the mistake of setting the rules more strictly than you can manage, the best thing to do is to stop the sadhana and immediately replace it by a new sadhana with a more achievable set of rules. Continuing the sadhana after breaking the rules is only advisable if you feel confident that it will not happen again. After breaking the same rule twice, you should stop the sadhana and replace it by a new sadhana with more humble objectives.

Hindus believe that whoever does any kind of sadhana will be tested not only by himself or herself, but also by the gods. In the great Hindu epics, it is most often Kama, the deity of desire, who tries to break a person's sadhana by creating distraction through special objects of desire. While doing Rasa Sadhana unexpected things may happen, pleasant or unpleasant. We should embrace them in the knowledge that the gods only get involved when a sadhana is really fruitful and powerful. Whatever happens at that time, had to happen sometime. The fact that it happens during the sadhana is a gift, because if it had happened at another time, the result might have been a lot worse.

Thoughts, Words, and Actions

Mastering our thoughts is a lot more difficult than mastering our words and actions. One may limit a sadhana to words and actions to begin with. But the Rasa will never be mastered if our thoughts are not mastered and it is often easier to attack the Rasa at the root, the original thought. Within the Hindu concept of karma, there is no difference between thinking about a bad thing and doing it.

Thoughts are always linked with the electrical processes in the computer that is our brain, while feelings are a kind of biochemical awareness felt in and through the body, which a computer does not have. Thinking and feeling are two sides of the same coin. We cannot master our feelings without mastering our thoughts and vice versa.

Mastering our thoughts is a gradual process. It is often best to adopt absolute rules regarding words and actions, while seeing the rules related to thoughts as absolute only with regard to prolonged thought. So, for example, if an angry thought comes in Anger Sadhana, it should immediately be replaced with countering thoughts. In Humor Sadhana, a serious thought should immediately be ridiculed. The thoughts that do not fit the sadhana will gradually subside, until by prolonged exercise we can get rid of them completely. Desirable neural and biochemical patterns take time to create and undesirable ones take even more time to be removed.

Rasa Sadhana is not about suppressing emotions! When we experience that a negative feeling keeps coming back, keeps festering inside, then we are on the wrong track in our Rasa Sadhana. Negative thoughts and emotions must be allowed sufficient inner expression for their origin to be properly analyzed. It is this very analysis, which emphasizes the witnessing factor, that may dissolve them. Just as thoughts will disappear when we look at them from a distance in meditation, emotions will disappear when we fearlessly challenge their very nature and origin.

The stricter the rules of a sadhana are set, the more important it becomes to control our feelings through body chemistry. Controlling sensory input and food quality on a daily basis are the only ways to make it happen. For example, to avoid angry thoughts altogether the body must be kept sufficiently cool all the time. To avoid worries the blood sugar levels should be stabilized, and so on.

Including special practices such as pranayama or worship in our daily routines is also very important for successful performance of prolonged Rasa Sadhana. Mastering the breath is essential in all Rasa Sadhana, so breathing exercises are always helpful. Exercises in positive thinking, such as doing daily worship of the deity who particularly relates to the Rasa (see chapter 18), are beneficial. Studies conducted at the Cleveland Clinical Foundation and Chester College (Professor David Smith) demonstrated that consciously and realistically imagining weightlifting exercises seriously increases muscle mass and power. If positive thinking can have such profound effects on the body, the potential for affecting our instinctive reactions, neural patterns, and biochemical balance with Rasa Sadhana must be equally extraordinary.

Lifelong Rasa Sadhana

A particular Rasa Sadhana can be adopted for a long period or even for a lifetime. After doing a sadhana for a modest time period, we may feel good about it and so strongly identify with the sadhana that we adopt it permanently.

As for the disagreeable Rasas, we may indeed feel that life is better without them. Disgust leads nowhere, so it is a most likely candidate for a lifelong sadhana. Anger may have its uses in communication, but even then, we may come to feel that in Anger we always lose more than we gain. Fear may give us warnings, but the one who is really fearless needs no warnings.

An agreeable Rasa may feel so good and right that we desire nothing else. We may spend all of our life in art, beauty, and decoration. Alternatively, we may be so absorbed in the miracle of life that nothing else makes sense. It is also possible to do a lifetime sadhana of an agreeable Rasa but limit it someway or other as needed to make that possible, as explained for various Rasas in Part 2.

Some people may perform a particular Rasa Sadhana as long as it takes to achieve the power or siddhi that comes along with it. The scriptures are quite clear, however, that such powers will eventually be lost if the sadhana is not maintained.

16

Balancing Sensory Input

If one cannot stop sensory input, choose
delicately at least.

Except in the states of sense withdrawal such as deep sleep, deep meditation, or coma, we continuously receive a large amount of information from our environment through the five senses: sight, sound, touch, smell, and taste. Most of this information is processed unconsciously and information molecules play a major role in that process.

At the locations where information transfers to the senses, very high concentrations of receptors for neurotransmitters are found. These information molecules filter the sensory pulses on their way to the brain. Sensory perception also strongly affects the concentration of information molecules throughout the body. It has been demonstrated, for example, that soothing sounds and sights may increase serotonin levels in the body. Harsh noise or a bad taste in the mouth may increase the levels of adrenalin. The senses are real hotspots for the transfer of emotional information. In waking consciousness, emotions and sensory input influence each other all the time.

Both the quality and quantity of information molecules in the body strongly relate to our earlier experiences, from childhood up to how the present day began. At each moment, our body contains a biochemical information pattern that colors the transfer of sensory input. All of our senses become very personal in this way.

Neurotransmitters are not only produced by the nerve cells of the brain. Many are also produced throughout the body by other nerve cells, white blood cells, cells of various organs such as the kidneys or the intestines, and so on. The entirety of neurotransmitters and receptors spread throughout the body is sometimes regarded as a sixth sense, which likewise affects our emotions and thoughts.

Avoiding Confusion

Lack of concentration causes many undesirable moods. If we are not centered, then things become confusing and confusion leads to Fear, Sadness, Anger, and Disgust. When we get too many options, like in a supermarket, our mind becomes confused and we become impossible to satisfy.

The extreme sensory input that is typical in modern society is highly confusing. While most people remain unaware of it, television brings people and scenes into our homes that we would never accept in our lives. The low-quality entertainment produced by the mass media is made more interesting by being spiced with rapidly changing images and sounds as well as scenes of sex and violence. As a result such entertainment produces Anger, Disgust, Fear, and Sadness. These disagreeable emotions make people so confused that they become completely addicted to intense sensory input. If the eyes, taste buds, ears, nose, or skin are not continuously receiving information that attracts the attention, confusion surfaces and becomes unbearable. While modern commerce can only sustain itself by increasingly stimulating our senses, we remain free to join this frenzy or not.

Practicing Calmness through withdrawal of the senses is essential. Focus means involvement and attachment, so the moment we focus on something, we become involved with and attached to it. Thus in order to get our Rasas under control we not only need to do some television-fasting and media-fasting, but also need to stop the continuous process of evaluating whether impressions are agreeable or not. This is the only way to stop attachment. When both the absorption and evaluation of impressions are brought to a halt, that enables the negative traces of earlier impressions to surface in a natural manner, allowing them to be properly treated by our intellect. Even when we are sincerely practicing Calmness, some sensory input may be unavoidable; that input should be consciously ignored. This is the true meaning of *pratyahara* or "withdrawal of the senses," one of the eight limbs of Ashtanga Yoga (see chapter 22).

On the other hand, certain sensory experiences can create subtle substances that nourish the mind. Sensory input can be used as a highly valuable tool to control the Rasas, but in order to work that way it must be used in a moderate fashion, with the focus on the best available quality. Positive sensory input is mostly valuable in changing a mood or in subtly sustaining one.

When the focus is directed inside or toward calming, uniform, and positive sensory input, the effect of disturbing sensory input from the environment can be reduced to a mere fraction. Even on a hectic street, there may be a beautiful little flower growing in between some concrete slabs and inner mantra recitation is always an available option.

The art of affecting our feelings through the senses is so broad that many, many books can and have been written on various aspects of it. In the following short sections, we merely take a peek at the subject.

Sound

In Indian philosophy, the creation of the phenomenal world proceeded from subtle to gross, that is, the five elements arose from the five *tanmatras*. "Tanmatra" literally means "only that" (*tan* = that, *matra* = only). Although their names are "sound, touch, sight, taste, and smell," these tanmatras are not the five senses as we know them, but pure frequencies or essences of the senses that preceded the creation of the phenomenal world.

Sound was the first manifestation of creation. This is similar to the Christian view of creation in which "God first created sound and the sound was God." For Hindus, this primordial sound is AUM. Out of sound was born the element of akasha (ether, void), and the other tan-matras and elements arose in turn:

❖ Akasha from Sound
❖ Air from Touch
❖ Fire from Sight
❖ Water from Taste
❖ Earth from Smell

Sound is the most powerful of the senses in controlling our Rasas, as it produces vibration in all five elements and therefore affects both body and consciousness. Sounds carry emotions and may release them.

Through the ears, sound directly generates many different kinds of neurotransmitters and other information molecules. The effect of sound in the body goes far beyond its sensory organ; it affects molecular vibra-tion throughout the body, determining the levels of order and chaos in molecular patterns. Information molecules and their receptors are in a continuous state of vibration, so the rhythm of music or mantras directly affects their linking potential. Sound also directly affects electrical trans-mission in nerve cells. Thus it is not surprising that music played in the intensive care departments of hospitals has been shown to heavily reduce patients' needs for tranquilizers.

Some sounds are known to have particularly positive and calming effects, such as the sounds of running water, of leaves being touched by the wind, of waves crashing on the seashore. Other sounds and espe-cially loud chaotic sounds of blenders, vacuum cleaners, traffic, and so on may increase stress, irritation, and nervousness.

A big advantage of modern times is that portable music players, car stereos, and computers can provide us with the music of our choice at almost any time. They can help to shut out negative impressions. But we should watch out for the radio: even a favorite radio station may trigger emotions that are not appropriate at a particular moment.

Memory plays an important role in the power of songs. People often get very positive feelings from hearing the songs that were their favorites in adolescence. Even if those songs sound harsh to others, they may produce very fine feelings in those who remember good times through them. Couples very often have one song that particularly reminds them of their first or best moments together.

Making music ourselves has the most powerful effect on our emotions because it forces us to completely focus on the sounds being created. When we are just listening to music our mind too easily wanders and, without full attention, the sound has less effect. For those who are musicians, playing music is probably the best way to change a mood. Singing or chanting produces the strongest vibrations throughout the body.

Singing a song inside is something done quite unconsciously by almost everybody. Unfortunately, many people feel ashamed about it and try to stop it when they detect it. Whether it is song or a mantra, it can help one to stay in a particular mood and stops the mind from wandering off in a variety of directions.

Mantra chanting in particular creates vibrations that produce prana and akasha. Chanted mantras are "postures" for the mind that can profoundly alter its emotional patterns. Indian philosophy speaks of the *mantra purusha,* the "person of sound;" this person, represented by the Sanskrit alphabet, impacts all parts of the body. Specific characters of the Sanskrit language work through the *marmas,* pressure points similar to those used in Japanese *shiatsu* or reflexology. A good example can be seen in the Gayatri Mantra (see the Conclusion of this book), which contains twenty-four syllables. Between them, they work on the entire body. The mantra AUM (pronounced OM) is the essence of all mantras. It represents cosmic consciousness, beyond words or concepts. AUM is the primordial sound of timeless reality that opens our innermost being to the vibrations of a higher reality; it is also a symbolic word for the perfect, the infinite, and the eternal, as well as the origin of all creation.

Touch

The sense of touch is strongly linked to the endorphins, the body's own morphine. When making love, the levels of endorphins in our blood may become two hundred times higher than normal.

Massage can work miracles as well, but the production of endorphins is only one aspect of it. Emotional stress is stored in the body and massage can release it. Proper handling of the pressure points directly affects the production of neurotransmitters.

Many sportsmen and women know the phenomenon of "runner's high," produced by physical exercise and involving a similar release of emotional stress from the body as well as the production of specific neurotransmitters like dopamine.

A world famous experiment on depressed monkeys showed that allowing them simple physical contact with other monkeys strongly increased their number of receptors for the anti-depressant neurotransmitter called CRF (Cortical Releasing Factor). The contact allowed them to escape from their depression through body chemistry. The experiment concluded that "hugs not drugs" should be used to deal with mental problems. Regularly hugging our partners, children, and friends creates a biochemical basis for feeling happy.

Cold and heat strongly affect blood circulation, breath, and heartbeat. If we feel cold, then this creates nervousness. Feeling hot for a short period is very relaxing but when the heat endures, it creates lethargy and increases irritability.

Sight

Colors have strong emotional value. Experiments with animals have shown that they can affect the production of neurotransmitters. The emotional value of colors is quite personal and depends on circumstances. However, generally speaking, soft, warm, and deep (composed) colors create the most positive emotions. Orange, red, and yellow are more stimulating and energizing (rajasic), while blue and green are more calming and inspiring (sattvic), and grays and other dark colors are more depressing and worrying (tamasic). Mixtures of sattvic and rajasic colors are generally best to keep around oneself. Bright colors increase tejas, our inner radiance.

Indian art uses specific colors to produce specific moods:

COLOR	RASA
Green	Shringara (Love)
White	Hasya (Joy)
Light-brown	Veerya (Courage)
Yellow	Adbhuta (Wonder)
Grey	Karuna (Sadness)
Red	Raudra (Anger)
Black	Bhayanaka (Fear)
Dark Blue	Vibhatsa (Disgust)

Shapes also affect our emotions. Rounded and harmonious shapes are more peace giving and inspiring (sattvic), while sharp shapes are more exciting and capturing (rajasic), and imbalanced shapes more confusing (tamasic).

The art of shapes and colors is beautifully expressed in the creation of yantras, geometrical patterns that express and provoke the energy patterns of particular Hindu deities. Meditation on these yantras may change the mind as profoundly as mantras can. Using mantra and yantra together engages both the verbal and visual sides of the brain and can work miracles for our emotional health.

The art of bringing harmony to our homes is equally powerful. Like Feng Shui, the Indian art of placement known as Vastu identifies the best shapes and colors to use in the construction of home and work environments. Vastu also takes into account many other aspects, such as the four directions, the location of water elements, the choice of indoor and outdoor plants, ventilation, and so on.

Nature provides us with refreshing and inspiring sights, which should be sought out as much as possible. Our work environments and especially our cities are usually deficient in the quality of colors and shapes. Grays and rectangular shapes are predominant. Architects of homes, buildings, and cities bear a responsibility that few really seem to appreciate. Keeping the eyes down is the best way to travel through most cities, because of their ugliness and the lack of positive stimuli. Very often street advertising stands out with plenty of color and beautiful pictures. We should be aware, however, that such displays are designed to increase our levels of desire (see chapter 25).

Of all senses, sight is the easiest one to shut down. Whenever rest is needed, we can shut our eyes for a minute and peace will be automatically generated through the production of melatonin.

Taste

As noted earlier, one of the translations for the word *rasa* is "taste." From the tanmatra of taste the water element is created, which is the primary element that affects the Rasas. That makes taste a very important sense when dealing with our emotions.

Food chemicals that come in contact with the taste buds of our tongue directly produce a variety of neurotransmitters. Eating sweets, for example, immediately increases the level of endorphins—our natural painkiller—in our body. That explains why a little sweet is very effective in soothing a hurt child.

Tastes also strongly relate to memories. Tastes that trigger agreeable and less agreeable memories will produce information molecules that create corresponding emotions. Personal body chemistry and temperament will also affect the production of information molecules through taste.

If we feel an unusual desire for a particular taste then it is the corresponding emotional effect that we are after. In most cases, it is fine to give in to it, as long as these desires do not become addictions. The bitter taste is calming and detaching, the pungent taste motivating and alerting, the salty taste sedating and grounding, while the sweet taste is soothing.

Addictions to the tastes of chocolate, coffee (caffeine), meat (adrenalin, dopamine), sugar (endorphins), fats (endorphins), and so on are based on the same basic problem as that of real "drugs": doses that are too high reduce our own ability to generate the related information molecules naturally, thus creating a dependency on the related taste and a need for ever higher doses.

The effect of the sense of taste goes far beyond the direct sensory level. It is unusual to taste something without eating it, so what we taste also affects our emotions through digestion. The best possible example is chocolate. The extremely strong attraction that many people experience toward chocolate is easily explained because it contains or produces serotonin (antidepressant), phenylethylamine (the "love peptide"), and endorphins as well. If eaten in relatively large quantities, the agreeable feelings that are generally produced through the taste are rapidly replaced by the less agreeable feelings that are caused by the high intake of sugar and fat and by a mildly toxic effect on the liver.

Sugars especially cause emotional imbalance through the insulin trap: Insulin is produced in the blood to even out our blood sugar levels. When the body detects extremely high sugar levels in the blood, the insulin reaction is so strong that our blood sugar level becomes too low, causing a new craving for sugar. When the blood sugar level is below the limits, it creates depression. If too high it causes hyperactivity. Eating too much sugar thus creates manic-depressive cycles of behavior.

Children especially need sweets now and then. It pays to remember that it is the soothing taste that they are really after. Choosing lollipops and hard candies that take a long time to dissolve is a smart way to avoid overloading their biochemistry with the sugars and fats contained within sweets.

The effect of foods through digestion is further discussed in chapter 17.

The taste of rotting foods in between the teeth is quite disgusting and creates feelings of disgust as well. Regular tooth brushing and flossing thus not only serves the health of our teeth, but also our emotional health.

Smell

According to evolution theory, smell is the most primitive sense. We have less power over the effect of smells on our feelings than over the other senses because there is only one synapse between the nerve that comes out of the nose and the amygdala in the brain. The amygdala, in turn, is able to affect body chemistry directly, without interference of our frontal brain, where our more conscious thinking takes place. That makes it very difficult to protect ourselves from the effects of intense smells on our body chemistry.

Thus we need to be aware of the emotional impact of bad smells in our environment. Modern hygiene has mostly eliminated the noxious smells of rotting waste in cities, but they have been replaced by those of the exhaust gases from traffic and factories. It is equally important to realize that bodily cleanliness affects our moods. Smells of our body and clothes may be rather subtle, but they are around all the time. Regular bathing and changing clothes is a logical practice.

The use of smells to positively affect moods is very old, from the use of incense to the wearing of perfumes and the perfuming of fabrics. In the devotional practices of Bhakti Yoga, smells become a symbol for the divine when scented objects such as flowers or incense are offered to the deity.

In modern aromatherapy the scents of essential oils are directly used to enhance well-being. Bergamot, sage, cedar, rose, sandalwood, and lavender have calming and soothing effects. Juniper, peppermint, and rosemary are more stimulating, a typical dopamine effect. As scents have very personal emotional effects, we can all easily be our own aroma therapists. Beware, however, of synthetic perfumes that might have adverse side effects, as smelling includes inhalation.

Beyond the Senses

Various energetic effects on the body and mind are still regarded as irrelevant by most scientists. Nevertheless, recent research shows many body-related energies that cannot be easily set aside: Electrical fields generated by body organs, magnetic brain waves and other magnetic fields, light and heat emissions by body cells and organs, structural coherence in the crystallization of fluid molecules, molecular vibrations, and more.*

It has, for example, been demonstrated that the recognition of a specific hormone by a receptor depends on resonant vibratory interactions between these molecules, comparable to the interactions of tuning forks. Another example lies in the importance of the depolarization and repolarization of the cell membranes in interaction with neurotransmitters in synapses. And of course, nerves use electrical currents in communication, which may logically be affected by electromagnetic energies, just like any other electrical current.

As long as science provides no conclusive information on this subject, we should be careful of contact with the many types of energy waves created by modern appliances, from cellular phones to high-tension power lines.

---

*Recommended reading: James L. Oschman, *Energy Medicine* (Edinburgh, U.K.: Harcourt Publishers Limited, 2000).

17

Cooking Emotions

Foods feed both matter and mind.

The Rasa Dhatu

The seven dhatus are the principal constituents of the body, literally the "body tissues." They need nourishment and give form to the physical body. Rasa as plasma or "nutritive juice" is the most essential dhatu that is derived from food, and all other dhatus are derived from it:

- ❖ Rasa (plasma) derived from the essence of food.
- ❖ Rakta (blood) derived from the essence of Rasa.
- ❖ Mamsa (flesh) derived from the essence of Rakta.
- ❖ Medha (fat) derived from the essence of Mamsa.
- ❖ Asthi (bones) derived from the essence of Medha.
- ❖ Majja (marrow) derived from the essence of Asthi.
- ❖ Shukra (semen) derived from the essence of Majja.

The plasma is the watery solution that carries the free chemicals in our blood, among which are the neurotransmitters and many substances that affect neurotransmitter activity. The science of Ayurveda regards plasma as both the carrier of essential nourishment and the promoter of happiness. Tantrics call the dhatu Rasa "the Juice of Love." When it starts "drying up," due to aging and also from living a less joyful life, our health starts to suffer and we need more moisture or juice in the body to remain healthy and happy. Thus good food is essential for our happiness.

Different food systems have different views on food balance. The Western food approach is mostly based on balancing proteins, fats, starches, vitamins, and minerals. The macrobiotic diet mostly balances female and male energies in food as yin and yang. Ayurveda mostly balances gunas, doshas, and tastes.

All these food systems create a balance of some kind, though the quality of that balance may be different. Even within food systems different kinds of balances can be created, serving different body types and lifestyles. Householders need more active energy so their food balance will need to be more rajasic, while that of saints may be more sattvic.

Balanced Ayurvedic Foods

According to Ayurveda, foods affect our emotions through the direct effect of taste (rasa), through the effect during digestion (virya), and the effect after digestion (vipaka). As explained in chapter 2 the resulting doshas and gunas stimulate the occurrence of particular Rasas. Understanding the effect of foods on doshas and gunas offers a great help in cooking foods that balance our Rasas.

Ayurveda also categorizes foods according to six principal tastes and teaches that any meal should contain all tastes in proper proportion. If they are not balanced, those who are eating the meal will remain chemically dissatisfied. The resulting emotional desire for a particular taste typically leads to overeating. Generally speaking, the sweet taste is the most needed; sour, pungent, and astringent tastes are needed in moderation; salty and bitter tastes are needed in small amounts only. This also depends on climate and personal biochemistry.

The direct effect of taste relates to particular gunas and doshas:

TASTES, GUNAS, AND DOSHAS

Taste	Example	Main Gunas	Dosha Increased Through Taste
Sweet	Honey	Sattva	Kapha
Sour	Lemon	Rajas	Pitta and Kapha
Salty	Salt	Rajas	Pitta and Kapha
Pungent	Black pepper	Rajas and Tamas	Vata and Pitta
Bitter	Coffee	Rajas	Vata
Astringent	Pomegranate	Rajas	Vata

However this overview only relates to the effect before digestion; the total effect of foods with a particular taste may be quite different from that shown in this table.

The effect during digestion (virya) is either hot or cold. Foods are also classified as dry or unctuous and as light or heavy. The effects of foods after digestion (vipaka) are classified as sweet, sour, or pungent. For some schools of Ayurveda, vipaka refers to categorizations of light or heavy. The vipaka effects are mostly important for foods that are used in excess over a long period. Through vipaka, addictions to certain foods and tastes lead to disturbance of the doshas.

On an energy level, the quality of foods is expressed through the resulting gunas. Tamasic foods (such as meat or old foods) are difficult to digest and contain little subtle energy and many toxins. They increase the related Rasas Fear and Disgust. Rajasic foods (such as rice and wheat) bring a lot of energy without being too difficult to digest and contain fewer toxins. They increase the related Rasas Love, Joy, Courage, Wonder, Sadness, and Anger. Sattvic foods (such as fruits and nuts) bring a lot of subtle energy, are very easily digested and very fresh and pure. They are the best basis for the Shanta Rasa and also stimulate the higher expressions of the other Rasas. If little physical labor is needed (requiring rajas), then they are the best possible food.

This subject is so broad that it fills many books, so we have only mentioned the main aspects. Further reading in *Ayurvedic Healing Cuisine* by Harish Johari* is advised for those who would like to implement Ayurvedic knowledge in their cooking. In addition to many great recipes, it contains overviews of many food types and their main effects.

Avoiding Emotionally Toxic Foods

Some foods may have toxic effects on our emotional well-being. This is a very diverse subject and in Western science little is known about many of these effects.

Meat is emotionally toxic primarily because it contains large amounts of neurotransmitters created by the fear and pain of the dying animal. These neurotransmitters increase blood pressure, muscle tension, and sugar conversion. Meat from animals that were killed in slaughterhouses—where they smelled blood and death in advance of their own death—is more toxic than meat from animals killed with less warning on a farm. The use of tranquilizers in animals, especially prior to their transport and slaughter, is particularly worrying. Red meat is to be avoided in particular because the biochemistry of mammals is the closest to our own. If you enjoy thinking and feeling like a scared pig, then please eat it.

Eating organic foods is another way to avoid emotionally toxic substances. Everybody knows that pesticides are unhealthy by nature, but few relate them to disturbed emotions. Dioxin is known to reduce emotional responses by reducing receptor activity. Organophosphates, a widely used group of pesticides, are known to affect the nervous system and may cause irritability at low doses. Many pesticides have hormone-like effects and are known to cause sex changes in water animals. What a pesticide disguised as the female estrogen hormone does to our emotional life remains uncertain. That an effect will be present seems only logical. Other pesticides are known to cause memory problems, depression, tiredness, headaches, and a reduction of intellectual capacities.

---

*Harish Johari, *Ayurvedic Healing Cuisine: 200 Vegetarian Recipes for Health, Balance, and Longevity* (Rochester, Vt.: Healing Arts Press, 2000).

All this information has only become available by coincidence through research that had bodily health as its subject. Research directly focused on the mental effects of pesticide residues would probably provide even more evidence of the relevance of organic foods for emotional health.

Some specific foods can be seen as emotionally toxic, because they may strongly unbalance our emotions. Refined sugars are a good example, because they increase serotonin and cause the depletion of subtle energy resources (see chapter 16, under "Taste"). Drinks that have high levels of caffeine are equally to be avoided or used in moderation because they increase the Fear Rasa. Coffee and tea are the most obvious examples, but colas and other caffeinated sodas and energy drinks are also a problem. A can of caffeinated soda holds about the same amount of caffeine as a cup of coffee. While adults are usually reserved in giving coffee to children, kids are often allowed to drink enormous amounts of caffeinated soda. Moreover, the effect of caffeine directly relates to body weight. Hyperactive children are the obvious result.

Avoiding strongly refined and old foods is equally important. These foods contain more toxins than fresh foods and very little vital energy, as prana or vitamins and minerals. Minerals and vitamins are essential in the production of most information molecules. It has been demonstrated, for example, that a magnesium deficiency reduces neurotransmitter activity. The brain itself is continuously flooded with blood, and blood chemistry strongly affects the way it functions. There is no doubt that junk foods make people unhappy. They cause feelings of boredom, sadness, and fatalism, followed by irritation, worry, and even anger as life catches up with them. For maintaining positive emotions, freshly prepared foods are a must.

Digestibility of Foods

Drowsiness, constipation, acidity, and so on are just the most obvious and extreme symptoms of disturbed digestion. These all too common symptoms clearly cause us to feel rather badly. However, less obvious digestion problems also affect our emotional well-being. Bad digestion means that many toxins are being produced inside the intestines. The organs of the digestive system are heavily loaded with receptors as well as production centers for information molecules that affect our emotions without our being conscious of it.

Foods and snacks that contain high levels of protein, fats, and refined sugars, such as many candy bars, are very difficult to digest. The digestion of meat always happens through a putrification process that creates high levels of toxic purines. Vegetarian foods as well as fresh milk products are digested through a much healthier process of fermentation.

Vegetarians must also watch out for digestion problems. While meat eaters need lots of fibers, vegetarians get enough of them easily, so they should avoid getting too much of them because they may irritate the intestines. Beans and vegetables that produce a lot of gas (vata) in the intestines must be prepared in such a way as to avoid it. The yogic diet contains plenty of raw foods because they provide the most prana. But when we do not regularly exercise like a yogi does, eating too many raw foods may cause vata problems. Yogis also mostly eat sattvic foods, in relatively small amounts. Some specific vegetarian foods are rather difficult to digest, such as many vegetarian meat substitutes (except if freshly prepared), mushrooms, celery, onions, garlic, and pasta.

The digestibility of foods can be strongly improved by the use of specific herbs and spices. Ginger, fennel, fenugreek, asafetida *(hing)*, and oregano are just a few examples of tasty spices that stimulate the production of saliva in the mouth and acids in the stomach, while reducing the production of gases in the intestines. A full description of the effect of the most common Indian spices can be found in Harish Johari's *Ayurvedic Healing Cuisine* book mentioned earlier.

Mood Foods

"Mood foods"—foods that have particular effects on the emotions—are becoming more and more popular. Some foods are more relaxing, others more stimulating. There is nothing wrong with eating in accordance with this approach as long as it is applied honestly and in moderation.

Ayurvedic knowledge regarding the effects of specific foods may be used to control specific Rasas, keeping in mind that such an approach is absolutely secondary to eating properly balanced food.

In India, for example, saffron deserts are very often made for special celebrations, because saffron creates a merry mood. When the guests depart, the people who remain behind will chew cardamom seeds in order to cool down the emotions and reduce the sadness of departure.

Each cook can help the people who eat his or her foods by subtly giving them the Rasa energies that they need at a particular moment. Spices not only provide taste to the food or aid in its digestion. Their high essential oil content also gives more taste (rasa) to life, though they should be properly used in accordance with personal constitution and circumstances.

Related to mood foods are certain rejuvenating agents called *rasayana* in Ayurveda. They mostly consist of specially treated metals, minerals, and precious stones.* The Rasa Shastra is the branch of Ayurveda that studies this art. The transmutation of basic metals into noble ones is called the Rasa Vidya or the science of mercury or alchemy.

The information about the body-mind link now being provided by Western science makes it clear that it is possible to abuse mood foods and even become addicted to them, so they need to be used with care (see chapter 25).

Other Aspects

Many other aspects of food preparation affect our health and emotions, such as how it is prepared and eaten, the compatibility of foods, different needs for different seasons and climates, and last but not least the mood of the cook. All these are fully explained in Harish Johari's book on Ayurvedic cuisine mentioned earlier.

---

*More information on the use of gem powders can be found in Harish Johari, *The Healing Power of Gemstones* (Rochester, Vt.: Destiny Books, 1996).

18

Daily Routines

Good and bad habits are easy to
develop and hard to lose.

Daily rituals develop and maintain positive emotions and thoughts. Daily habits are not only needed to regulate the lives of children, but also to bring order to the childlike mind of any adult. They keep us in tune with the natural cycles and help to create and broaden the right neural and biochemical patterns on a regular basis without our needing to think about it. If we do everything in a different way every day then we have to think about it all the time. This leaves us less time and energy to get the benefit from what we are doing. Above all, repetition is a key element in changing our neural and biochemical patterns.

Daily rituals are a part of our sadhana and work in the same way: We follow them because we promised ourselves to do so—no questioning needed. As our personality changes we can adapt them, but only now and then.

When faced with the following guidelines for maintaining emotionally healthy daily routines, many may despair. Daily routines are just one part of the many things we feel we should do to live a good life, so it is only natural that the task seems overwhelming at times. The discrepancy between knowing and doing can be a cause of severe emotional distress. It may lead to Disgust, Sadness, and Fear and thus it can be a real obstacle in Rasa Sadhana. If we feel that this discrepancy is causing real problems, then we should do Duty Sadhana. Doing Duty Sadhana means that for a period we live as perfectly as we know how, starting with one day or more and then gradually building on that. That day or week we will definitely wake up before sunrise, eat only balanced food, watch only the really interesting things on television, and live according to all the other do's and don'ts that we believe apply to us. Anybody can do this for a day and that is enough to begin with. This sadhana is not about being impossibly perfect or about living the life of a saint for a day or so, but about being as perfect as we can reasonably achieve, depending on the situation.

Doing such sadhana removes the dissatisfaction regarding our inability to live up to our expectations. Even after the sadhana is done, we can remain satisfied with ourselves because we know that we can do it for a short period and that we will do it again for ever longer periods. We are working on it, so there is no reason to feel bad about our imperfections. Combining such sadhana with a gradual, permanent integration of healthy daily routines in life is a very powerful approach.

While following one's daily routines, it is extremely important to listen to the needs of the body as well and not suppress its natural functions. Never hold back on urination, defecation, vomiting, sneezing, belching, and yawning.

Daily routines are a very broad subject that we can only briefly touch, concentrating on some of the main aspects. Many more valuable details are found in the *Dhanwantari* book by Harish Johari.*

Tuning into Natural Cycles

According to Kundalini Yoga† energy moves in regular patterns through the chakras and the elements, but there is no particular pattern of the occurrence of Rasas. Still, the change of vital energies in the atmosphere

---

*Harish Johari, *Dhanwantari* (Rochester, Vt.: Healing Arts Press, 2001).

†For more information, see Harish Johari, *Chakras* (Rochester, Vt.: Destiny Books, 1998).

throughout the day also affects them. At some times of the day, certain Rasas will more easily dominate:

RASAS AND TIMES OF THE DAY

Time of Day	Dominating Rasas	Rasas to Stimulate
Dawn	Calmness, Love	Calmness, Love
Morning	Courage	Courage
Afternoon	Courage, Joy	Courage, Joy
Dusk	Sadness, Disgust, Anger, Fear	Calmness
Evening	Disgust, Anger, Fear	Love, Joy

At dawn, meditation comes very naturally and easily because the Shanta Rasa is predominant at that time. It is also a great time to experience Shringara in a refined way, enjoying and creating spiritual art and poetry, performing rituals or spending quality time with our loved ones.

In the morning we should undertake new tasks and tasks that require a lot of inner strength, because the Courage Rasa comes most naturally at that time. The afternoon is also good for doing work, but especially after the midday meal we should take some time to rest and enjoy good company and some laughter.

It is mostly at dusk and in the evening that the less desirable Rasas are likely to manifest. The time of dusk should be spent in meditation in order to prevent that. For the same reason, the evening is a good time for light entertainment and to enjoy the arts. In ancient days kings and rich people used to hire entertainers to brighten up every evening.

Waking Up

To bring our personal energy patterns into accord with the symphony of our solar system, getting up before sunrise is essential. At ninety minutes before dawn, a great surge of energy is released and repeats itself even stronger about thirty minutes before dawn. Scientists have found that this causes our blood to thin dramatically and infuses the entire body with new chemicals. Sanskrit scriptures call this the "time of the nectar of life." To ensure good health and vitality, both physical and emotional, it is extremely important that at that time the body has already discharged stool and urine. If not, all toxins and waste gases produced during the night will be recirculated in the system.

Early morning is the best time for the Shanta Rasa, so we should remain calm and light-hearted as much as possible, setting the right pattern for the coming day. Getting up early also means that we have the time to slowly let the system wake, instead of having to rush through the entire process to be in time for work.

Many beneficial things can be done in the early morning, of which sitting up straight (preferably without back support) is the most important because then gravity automatically helps the bowel movement. Concentrating on soothing colors, shapes, and sounds as well as taking a slow early morning walk are very good. Washing hands, teeth, and face with water just below room temperature should happen before sunrise as well, making sure the eyes are washed at the same time the teeth are cleaned.

The minutes before and during sunrise are the best time of day for meditation. At the exact moment of sunrise, the organism automatically breathes through both nostrils simultaneously, so that the energy can flow upward through the Sushumna Nadi. The left and right sides of the forebrain, the solar and lunar, male and female energies all become balanced automatically. People who try meditation for the first time at sunrise will be surprised by the ease with which the Calmness Rasa comes and how it may linger the rest of the day.

Bathing

As soon as thirty minutes after waking the morning bath can be started. It cures dullness and drowsiness, dissolves sorrow, creates elation, increases enthusiasm, and gives vital energy to the system. The water should be lukewarm and the body should be exposed to it step by step.

Temperature shocks are to be avoided. Bathroom singers and hummers are famous in India up to the point where one who does not sing in the bath is besieged by concerns about his or her health.

After the bath we should put on fresh clothes so as not to wear old vibrations and smells. Putting some oil on the hair prevents the loss of electrical energy, protects memory, and discourages fantasy.

Worship

Spiritual rituals (puja) create positive impressions that nourish the mind and strengthen our Rasas of preference. We can engage all the senses— through focusing on the icons of deities, lighting incense, ringing bells, and chanting mantras—in order to stimulate those Rasas and thoughts that we cherish. Spiritual worship of any kind strengthens the higher aspects of the Rasas of Calmness, Wonder, and Love inside us. The best time for spiritual rituals is the morning. They will be the most beneficial when performed while being clean inside and outside.

An image or yantra of a deity symbolizes the form or body of the deity, whereas the mantra of the deity symbolizes the mind, spirit, consciousness, or name. They enable us to get in contact with the energy patterns associated with the particular deity, with that specific divine aspect of God. Daily meditation on the deity associated with a particular Rasa—such as Krishna for Shringara (Love) or Yama for Bhayanaka (Fear)—helps one to awaken and purify that deity and the Rasa within oneself. Daily concentration on the courage and selfless service of Hanuman, for example, will make it that much easier to follow his example in time of need during the day. Both the mental image of Hanuman and the Hanuman mantra will act as carriers of that attitude. They can be visualized or recited at any time.

Meals

It is generally advisable to eat only two meals a day: a late breakfast and a large meal taken between noon and sunset, during the most rajasic time of the day.

In the morning sattvic energy is dominant, so we should concentrate on a light breakfast with easily digestible foods. Fruits, seeds, and nuts are best, but if you have to do a lot of physical labor, you should make sure to ingest sufficient gross energy. With exception sometimes for cold climates, breakfast should be taken after morning meditation, puja, and physical exercise, which all will be more fruitful on an empty stomach.

The large meal taken between noon and sunset should contain all necessary ingredients for good health. After the meal, we should take some time off so that the body may concentrate all energy on digestion. It is the best time to enjoy good company, jokes, and most hobbies.

In the evening the energy becomes more tamasic. If we still feel the need to eat at that time, we should try to make it a light meal, otherwise we will only increase tamas. It certainly should be eaten several hours before sleep.

These are general guidelines, but we should learn to listen to our own body also. When enough food has been ingested, our body sends corresponding signals to our brain. We should be careful not to ignore these signals and overload our system just for the sake of taste-enjoyment.

Exercise

If we refrain from daily body exercise we ignore the vital link between body and mind. Most mild physical exercises will infuse the body with pranic energy, release tensions hidden deep inside, improve circulation, and harmonize the breathing pattern. Thus the best possible basis is created for a happy day. Walking or running at moderate speed, deep breathing, yoga postures, rhythmic movements, and twisting are just some of the options. Exercises that cause exhaustion are best avoided except for specific purposes.

Hobbies

It is important to relax on a daily basis and do something without material or practical purpose. If meditation can be a daily hobby, that is the best. But many other hobbies are very valuable as well, such as gardening, taking care of pet animals, playing music, painting, and so on. When they are fully enjoyed they can help to strengthen one's Rasa of preference. Spending some leisure time is the best way to accept that some problems in life cannot be solved instantly. Life should be enjoyed.

Sleep

With exception for people who are ill, it is most important not to sleep during the day and certainly not after taking a meal. Sleeping during the day disturbs gases, bile, lymph, blood flow, and our natural sleeping rhythm. Sleep following a meal completely disturbs the digestion process and causes constipation.

Sleep is a natural process for rejuvenating the body and mind, but should happen in proper proportion. When we sleep for too long, the last few hours will no longer bring any deep sleep and will make us tamasic by increasing kapha. Then we remain constantly in the dream state, which consumes energy uselessly. If we awaken still feeling tired and drowsy, then most likely we have slept too long. We should gradually reduce the period of sleep until we start waking up feeling fresh and vitalized.

For those who have difficulty falling asleep, massaging the feet just before retiring is a sure cure. For everyone, it protects against disease. It is good to avoid covering the face while sleeping because doing so forces us to breathe in exhaled carbon dioxide, which diminishes the healthy intake of oxygen.

Never sleep with the feet pointing to the south: If the body is viewed as a magnet with the head equal to the North Pole and the feet equal to the South Pole, sleeping with the feet facing south disturbs the body magnet because like poles repel one another. It is preferable to sleep on the left side, so that the weight of the stomach won't compress the liver while we sleep. Sleeping on the left side also enhances the ease of breathing, freeing the right lung from any crowding by the heart.

19

Emotional Emergencies

*Find the one inside that is always watching
without being affected.*

There may be times when you are so absorbed by one of the less desirable Rasas that it feels dangerous. Anger, Fear, Sadness, or Disgust all can lead to a state where you may lose control and act in a regrettable way. Those are the times to open this book and turn to this chapter. The following steps will definitely aid you in regaining control.

Step 1: Stop Identifying with the Rasa

You are in charge; whatever you do is your responsibility and you always have the power to change your emotional state. Remember that whatever you may be feeling, it is nothing more than a temporary state of body and mind. Put any specific reasons for that state temporarily out of your mind—they are less important than your emotional health. Nothing that might have caused this state is reason enough for losing control. Whatever happened, the real you remains unaffected.

Step 2: Immediately Change Your Body Chemistry

Create the proper biochemical basis for changing the Rasa in just a few minutes. In case of:

❖ Anger: Take a relatively cold shower, drink several glasses of cool water, and chew some green cardamom seeds afterward. Wear a necklace of pearls or eat pearl powder if available. Stop eating food until the Anger is gone.

❖ Fear (Anxiety): Eat some fresh ginger and drink some lemon juice in water.

❖ Sadness: Do not hold back your tears—releasing them helps to release the sadness. Rinse the eyes afterward with cool water or rose water. Chew some fenugreek leaves and saffron or eat a light sweet dish that contains one or both of these spices.

❖ Disgust (Depression): Eat a good amount of fresh ginger and take some fruit juices as well.

For those who practice Swar Yoga,* immediately change nostril dominance in all cases of emotional emergency.

Step 3: Induce Calmness

Perform the relaxing, breathing, and meditation exercises that you are most comfortable with, in order to create Calmness as an intermediate state in changing toward a desirable Rasa.

If you have not yet learned any such exercises:

❖ Slow down your breath through the following exercise: Hold your breath for as long as you comfortably can, then breathe out slowly, breathe in and again hold your breath. Repeat this exercise until your breathing remains slow.

---

*For more information on Swar Yoga see: Harish Johari, *Breath, Mind, and Consciousness* (Rochester, Vt.: Destiny Books, 1989).

❖ Balance both sides of the brain through the exercise of alternate nostril breathing: Breathe in through the left nostril and breathe out through the right. Breathe in slowly through the right nostril and breathe out slowly through the left, and so on. Use the thumb to block the nostrils as needed (or, if you know this pranayama technique, use the proper hand posture).

❖ Exercise your witnessing consciousness: Sit quietly in a comfortable position and close your eyes while breathing slowly. Watch your thoughts but try not to get caught by them, do not feed them through association. Do not get nervous because they keep coming. It is all right that they come. Just watch them without studying them or thinking about them. Do this for as long as you are comfortable with it.

❖ Again repeat the first breathing exercise. When your mind starts wandering off too much, stop.

Do this Calmness exercise for no less than fifteen minutes, the longer the better.

Step 4: Focus on the Desirable Enemy Rasas

In all cases, seeking out one's loved ones and having a good time with them by enjoying some natural beauty, art, and light chatter together is the best way to change the unpleasant Rasa to the Rasas of Love, Joy, and Wonder. Refrain from discussing your problem until you really feel reasonably happy again.

If you have nobody to turn to at this time, seek out natural beauty and the arts and remember those who care for you, maybe by looking at their photographs, reading some old letters, and so on. Feel loved and be loving and kind to whatever you see or whomever you meet.

In many cases of emotional turmoil, you may not feel like joining with your loved ones. It is good, however, to have them around even if you have to make it clear to them that you prefer not to communicate. As long as you are in that state, practice Calmness.

In case of Fear and anxiety, a good way to strengthen the Courage Rasa is to practice any physical disciplines that you have already mastered, such as yoga postures, martial art, and various sports.

Step 5: Analyze the Problem

Now that the disagreeable Rasa has mostly gone, analyze the attachment that lies at the basis of the Rasa and detach yourself from it:

❖ Anger: Analyze the unfulfilled expectation that triggered it and tell yourself to stop expecting it.

❖ Fear: Analyze the threatened identification that caused it and tell yourself to stop identifying with it.

❖ Sadness: Analyze the suffering caused by ignorance that created it and teach yourself to see through illusion.

❖ Disgust: No analysis needed; just forget whatever disgusted you and proceed immediately to step 6.

Reading through the related chapter in Part 2 may also be of help. Now that you feel more detached from the desires that feed these Rasas, you might also try to analyze the particular problem and see if there is a way to avoid it. If a solution seems possible, plan how to bring it about. If the problem has no solution, accept it.

Step 6: Exercise Your Control

Following this step by step program is usually very beneficial, but once you calm down, you should also realize that becoming so upset indicates that you need to gain more control over the particular Rasa. To avoid getting caught by it again, set the conditions for a Rasa Sadhana of that Rasa.

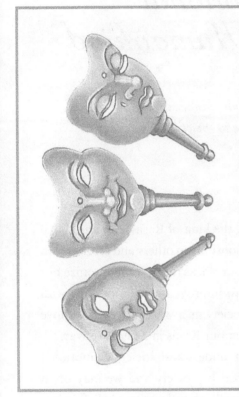

PART FOUR

Our Rasas in Society

20

The Emotional Evolution of Humankind

*Without inner peace, how can we dream
of bringing peace to society?*

As outlined in chapter 5 on Shringara, the king of Rasas, our emotional state is strongly influenced by our relationships to others and especially to our family and friends. To harmonize our Rasas means to harmonize our relationships. It is much easier for us to improve our relationships with those who are close to us than with society as a whole. Even if we love everyone, society can still strongly affect our Rasas in a negative way.

In mastering our Rasas we must understand society's emotional evolution. Our views on life are shaped by society and we may often find ourselves obstructed by our cultural inhibitions and beliefs when we work with the Rasas. In society, it is morality or the lack of it that creates agreeable or less agreeable Rasas. According to Hindu philosophy, dharma is the moral code of conduct that follows the laws of existence. *Sudharma* means to adopt the course of action best suited to one's place in society and one's path to liberation. Whether a course of action becomes moral or immoral largely depends on how it affects people's emotions. If our actions unnecessarily cause Sadness, Anger, or any of the other less agreeable Rasas, then they may well be immoral.

The History of Rasas in India

The earliest recorded use of the word "Rasa" is found in the Rig Veda, first of the early holy scriptures of Hinduism. Historians and scholars have most often interpreted the word "Rasa" in the Rig Veda as signifying: a river; an ocean that flows around the atmosphere and the world; a name of the earth goddess; or the juice of the *soma* plant. In the Atharva Veda it signifies juice squeezed from a grain. Nevertheless, many descriptions of the natural world given in the Vedas symbolize inner processes and elements, so Rasa may have had the same meaning in the Vedas as it certainly came to have at a later stage: "the essence of moods and emotions."

The word "Rasa" takes on a clearer meaning in later scriptures like the Upanishads, where it stands for "essence." In the Taittiriya Upanishad it gets an even more philosophical significance as the "essence of *ananda* (bliss)." *Sat* (truth), *chit* (consciousness), and ananda (bliss) are the three aspects of enlightenment and ananda in particular signifies the "feeling" aspect.

The Natya Shastra—written by the sage Bharata Muni in the fourth or fifth century CE—is generally recognized as the most important work on Rasas because it clearly defines eight of the nine Rasas. The principal theme of this book is the dramatic art. It describes the relationship between the literary and technical aspects of Rasas in a play, manifested through gestures, facial expressions, poetics, music, costumes, scene settings, and so on. It also stresses the need for an actor to learn philosophy and psychology, as they are essential for the successful portrayal of various Rasas.

The authorship of this work is somewhat unclear, because originally the word "bharata" meant "the actor of a drama." So it is quite possible that the treatise on the activities of *a* bharata was later attributed to a person named Bharata. The first verse calls it the "science of gesticulation and dance as originally imparted by the Hindu deity Brahma." The sixteenth verse names it the "Natya Veda" or fifth Veda, born out of the four Vedas and their ancillaries.

The seventeenth verse particularly associates the Rasas with the

Atharva Veda, named by some as the book of "the holy magic that brings happiness." Others call it a book of "black magic." The Natya Shastra contains about 5,600 verses, but the actual original composed by Brahma himself is supposed to have been 36,000 verses long.

Abhinavagupta, an eleventh century Kashmiri philosopher, introduced the ninth Rasa (Shanta), which was not originally included in Bharata's Natya Shastra, although in the ninth century Anandavardhana had already described the Shanta Rasa as the main Rasa of the Mahabharata.

It is quite astonishing that the Indian tradition managed to create a complete overview of these Rasas so long ago, while in Western science, Charles Darwin of the nineteenth century first became aware that people from all over the world recognize the same facial expressions as demonstrating particular emotions. In more modern times, Paul Ekmans made a study in twenty-one different cultures with photographs made of facial expressions and came to the conclusion that six basic emotions exist: Wonder, Fear, Anger, Joy, Disgust, and Sadness. Compared to the nine Rasas of Hinduism, his overview lacks Love, Calmness, and Courage, perhaps because these relate less clearly to facial expressions.

In any case, knowledge about the Rasas in Indian society is truly ancient. It has undoubtedly affected Indian society in all its aspects. The cultivation of agreeable Rasas has found expression especially in yoga and spirituality, Indian art and literature, social work and politics, family life and education, Ayurvedic therapy, and so forth. These subjects are outlined in further chapters.

Rasas in Modern Society

According to Hindu philosophy, we are now in the Kali Yuga, the "age of iron, conflict, ignorance, and darkness." The Kali Yuga leads up to the destruction of this world in preparation for a new creation and a new cycle of yugas. According to the Vishnu Purana—one of the oldest sacred texts of India—in Kali Yuga, "The leaders who rule over the Earth will be violent and seize the goods of their subjects. Moral values and the rule of the law (of dharma) will lessen from day to day until the world will be completely perverted and agnosticism (principal doubt) will gain the day among men."

If one evaluates the civilization level of modern society through the quality of its emotions and morality, one may indeed see it as going down. Historians might debate this question for ages, but the historical question is not very important. As the Kali Yuga is supposed to have started many thousands of years ago, it includes most of humanity's relatively well-known history. And today a majority of modern societies cultivate many of the less desirable Rasas and have completely lost touch with the finer expressions of the desirable Rasas. Modern mainstream culture sees egoism, cynicism, ambition, greed, gluttony, disgust, and so on as rather acceptable values, while higher values such as compassion, modesty, honesty, humility, and love are all too often rejected as naïve, inefficient, and hypocritical, and those who express them are seen as spineless losers.

There are many examples of this principal unhappiness that seems to have caught so many people in its grip. It is visible in the commonness of vulgar language, in the use of legal and illegal drugs, in the levels of crime and violence, in the instability of couples, families, and other relationships and in so many other ways. Some of these symptoms are discussed in the following chapters, so it seems best to leave it at that because it is really a sad story.

All people value the higher Rasas, but many remain largely unaware of doing so. For people who consciously value the higher Rasas, the emotional and moral state of society may be a cause of Anger, Sadness, Fear, and Disgust. But being caught by those feelings is obviously counterproductive. Truth is the only answer and the truth is that this rather sorry age is an illusion. First of all, this planet is only a grain of dust in the universe, so while we should do our share in caring for it out of our sense of dharma, what actually happens to it is of no consequence to the universe as a whole. Second, all problems and all suffering are opportunities for learning: The bigger the problem, the more advanced the lesson becomes. Hindu philosophy says that Kali Yuga offers humankind a rather advanced class in Bhakti Yoga. Third, for all bad things that happen, one good thing more than compensates. Many good things keep happening and are a part of the lesson just the same. Fourth, time itself is an illusion and so is Kali Yuga. Nothing lasts forever except truth.

The first responsibility that we have is to take care of ourselves. Only if we have the self-control to maintain the agreeable moods and a strict sense of morality (dharma) can we be of any real help to society. If we do not yet have such control, we should work on it and find people of like mind to be with. The majority of us suffer more from the lack of society's Love for us, rather than because of the suffering of society itself. In this age, shutting out the part of society that follows a different road is a necessity as long as that part causes any of the less desirable Rasas to catch us. Seeking out the people who are willing to give more than they take is the logical consequence.

If out of pity we want to reduce the suffering of this world (see also chapter 24), then we should have the Compassion to do so by spreading true knowledge. If we want to react in Anger to defend righteousness, we should first of all truly forgive and promote the truth of dharma without violence in thought, word, and deed. Acting out of Fear or Disgust should be avoided in any case.

21
Rasas and Western Science

Feeling happy is the best medicine that
laboratories may yet invent.

Effects of Emotions on Health

Negative emotional and thought patterns can certainly cause disease. There is a very strong connection between our emotional biochemistry and our immune system. Many viruses use the same receptors as our neurotransmitters in order to penetrate body cells. Positive emotions generate high levels of positive neurotransmitters in our body, which then occupy the receptors, effectively blocking the viruses from entering.

For example, the rhinovirus that causes the common cold uses the same receptor as noradrenalin, one of the neurotransmitters that is essential in feeling strong and cheerful. The feelings of Courage and Joy thus provide very good protection against the common cold because they reduce the number of available receptors for the rhinovirus.

Statistic research has also shown that people who are often caught by fear, aggression, and depression are twice as likely to develop asthma, arthritis, headaches, ulcers, and heart diseases. The scope of the health risk for heart diseases caused by negative emotions was found to be as high as that caused by smoking or high cholesterol levels.

Other important research in this field has focused on the herpes virus that remains forever in the body of a person who has had the disease. Through the production of antibodies in the blood, the activity level of the virus can be easily monitored. Research shows that the virus becomes more active in people under stress, such as students during examination periods, recently divorced couples, people with very ill family members, and so on.

Research also shows a clear relationship between Anger and cardiovascular diseases. A clear relationship has also been established between depression and the reduced capacity of the body to fight cancer cells or to heal more simple things like broken bones.

As more research is done on this subject, it will not be very surprising if humankind eventually comes to the conclusion that feeling unhappy is the most important cause of disease. Then society might be much more interested in actively promoting emotional well-being. People already fear disease as a cause of unhappiness—slowly they will come to realize that this relationship works both ways.

More Research Needed

Modern science has only recently begun to discover the relationship between the body and emotional well-being. An essential role in this evolution has been played by the research work of Candace B. Pert, whose discovery of endorphins as the body's own morphine was only the beginning of a brave struggle to demonstrate many body-mind links using traditional Western scientific methods. Her work is described for less scientific minds in the grand book *The Molecules of Emotion*.* The publication of the monumental work *Emotional Intelligence* by Daniel Goleman† has also dramatically altered public opinion on the importance of our emotional life, partially because of the vast amount of evidence presented in this work and partially through his clever demonstra-

---

*Candace B. Pert, Ph.D., *The Molecules of Emotion* (New York: Scribner, 1997).
†Daniel Goleman, *Emotional Intelligence: Why It Can Matter More than IQ* (New York: Bantam, 1995).

tion of the effects of emotional intelligence on business success, a sure way to catch attention these days.

The question remains: "What kind of research would be needed to bring more clarity on this subject to society? What future scientific findings might be valuable in understanding even better how to work with our Rasas?"

Technically speaking, a major breakthrough would consist of the development of detection techniques for neurotransmitters in the bodies of living people. Currently, apart from taking blood samples, most analysis on the presence of neurochemicals in human brains and other organs is done on dead bodies. Various tissues must be minced in order to detect the minute traces of neurotransmitters that affect our emotions. This is a lengthy process with questionable results, and one that causes a lot of suffering in laboratory animals when they are used as subjects. Fortunately, various types of brain scanning that focus on neurotransmitters are under development.

The greatest need is for science to come up with holistic research that brings real wisdom to the public and policy makers. It would be fairly easy, for example, to study the effect of meat on aggression in groups of people or monkeys. Likewise for the effect of grey versus bright colors in an environment, or the effects of various types of music, or comparisons of the effects of organic versus non-organic foods, old versus fresh foods, and so on. As modern society depends so strongly upon the opinion of science, such research would be a real gift.

Another interesting question for science is whether the nine Rasas can be recognized in biochemical patterns. Rasas are not purely biochemical, but it is probable that nine biochemical patterns correspond quite closely to the nine Rasas. Do the relationships of enmity, neutrality, and friendship between the Rasas also exist on a biochemical level? Such research would be very helpful in further research, therapy, and policy making.

Another important evolution of science would be to move beyond the purely biochemical level and enter the field of more subtle energies. There is so much uncertainty about this subject, which might well be far more important than the purely biochemical level. Such research might include electrical and magnetic fields, light and heat emissions, molecular vibrations, and so on. Today there is no clear scientific indication of the tantric notion that something called Rasa governs our moods and emotions as "a kind of energy that is neither purely physical nor purely mental, but partly physical and mental." However, not so long ago there was no scientific proof that moods and emotions had any counterpart in the body. While the physical aspect might today be described as "information molecules," the energetic aspect might one day be called "information energies."

Faulty Interpretation

All kinds of media currently bombard the public with fragmented information such as the claims that sugar is good for unhappy people, carrots cause depression, or meat is good for building confidence. Such information is often based on some new research indicating that one food or another creates an increase or decrease in a given neurotransmitter, which is related to a particular emotional pattern. This kind of information is very often created by clever marketing strategies (see chapter 25) and is best discarded.

As science discovers more electro-biochemical expressions of our thoughts and emotions, a tendency exists to use this information to degrade our feelings, thoughts, morality, and even spiritual experiences to a purely physical level. Some spiritual experiences are thus classified as "abnormal brain behavior, triggered by sensory deprivation and other techniques." Romance, artistic creativity, philosophy, and so on are thus all reduced to the illusionary deficiency of a burping electro-biochemical soup.

This kind of interpretation of scientific findings is completely faulty. Body and mind are just two sides of the same coin. If all our feelings and ideas are a product of our body, then logic dictates that the state of our body is just an expression of our thoughts and feelings as well. Desirable feelings go hand in hand with healthy body chemistry, while less desirable feelings are created by and create disturbed body chemistry. The one-sided approach to this duality is demonic in nature and makes us slaves of our bodies, but it remains very clear that we can be masters of our bodies, if we so choose. Science itself clearly shows how, for example, new neural patterns can be created and strengthened, allowing us to develop new thought patterns and emotional responses. Science may doubt whether yogic practices are able to create new paths that transcend normal levels of happiness, but if every such demonstration is classified as an anomaly or compared to a drug-like effect, science is not serving humanity as it should.

However, many scientists today are making a courageous and open-minded effort to properly interpret scientific facts on the body-mind link. Commerce and the mass media are much more guilty of faulty and ideological interpretation of these facts than science itself.

22

Rasas, Religion, Spirituality, and Yoga

Whether one yoga stands higher than another
is an entirely personal matter.

Rasa Yoga

The word "yoga" is derived from the Sanskrit root *yuj,* which means "to unite, to join, to add." The union in yoga, if considered at the gross physical level, is between the upper brain and the lower brain (the conscious with the subconscious) and between the left and right hemispheres (the solar and lunar energies). At a subtle level the union of yoga is between one's individual consciousness and cosmic consciousness. So yoga presents a system that creates a state of unification of mental processes and consciousness. Specific branches of yoga are based on particular disciplines and exercises through which this union of individual and cosmic consciousness may be obtained.

Rasa Sadhana really is Rasa Yoga. It is based on a set of disciplines with the objective of unifying our mental emotions (Bhava) with the essential fine sentiments or Rasas that are present in the Self, the individualized consciousness, the chitta (see chapter 4). Individual consciousness joins in cosmic consciousness when everything becomes divine Love and Beauty, when the illusion of duality causes only Joy, when knowledge instead of ignorance causes Wonder, when doubts have been replaced with effortless Courage, when ever-lasting Peace is attained. The Rasas are just one way to look at our being, next to many others like the chakras in Kundalini Yoga, the gunas in Ayurveda, or the basic instincts in Western psychology.

Rasa Sadhana relates to the worship of Shakti and of Vishnu as Krishna and is very much a part of the Hindu tradition and daily Indian life. According to the tantric tradition, life should be consciously enjoyed and our moods should also be enjoyed and enjoyable. This is contrary to the typical attitude of a sadhu, who concentrates on creating only one particular mood: Shanta or Calmness. Such an ascetic attitude is mostly seen in worshippers of the god Shiva.

Both the Shiva and Shakti traditions look at all of our needs and desires, our success in fulfilling them, and life itself as parts of the illusion that is called maya. The yogi rejects the illusion and searches for the truth inside: That which is never changing. The tantric choice lies in embracing the illusion without delusion, freely and consciously enjoying the game of life, leela.* In practice, most of the Hindu tradition is a mixture of both approaches, now withdrawing, then embracing. It is also a matter of personal choice and the evolution of consciousness.

Prolonged or lifelong Rasa Sadhana brings the special powers or siddhis that are described for each Rasa in Part 2 of this book. These supernatural powers are based on gaining absolute control over the elements. The very same siddhis are attainable in all other branches of yoga. For example, in Kundalini Yoga the powers of anima, laghima, mahima, prapti, prakam, vashitva, ishatattva, and bhukti become available by reaching the state of non-dual consciousness through prolonged meditation *(dhyana)* on the spiritual heart.[†]

Siddhis are only the by-product of sadhana, not the aim. As with

---

*More information on the concept of leela from the point of view of the chakras can be found in the book by Harish Johari, *Leela: The Game of Self-Knowledge* (Rochester, Vt.: Destiny Books, 1993). The book also contains an actual game board on which this chakras game can be played.

†For more information, see Harish Johari, *Chakras* (Rochester, Vt.: Destiny Books, 2000).

every yoga, the culmination of Rasa Yoga is enlightenment. But even if it only takes us halfway, it will already have earned the term "yoga."

Rasa Yoga can be a valuable part of any yoga tradition, just like Tantra Yoga contains Mantra Yoga, Hatha Yoga, Laya Yoga, and Raja Yoga. Most yoga techniques consume time, and householders in particular usually have no more than a few hours a day to spend on them, if they are lucky to have even that much freedom. Rasa Yoga can be performed twenty-four hours a day without consuming time, so it represents an ideal complementary exercise.

In the Vedic tradition, life is divided into four periods: *brahmacharya* (celibacy), *grihastha* (life of a householder), *vanaprastha* (withdrawal), and *sanyasa* (renunciation). Each period lasts twenty-five years on average. We can better understand the role of Rasa Yoga by looking at it in the context of these stages of life:

❖ The brahmacharya period starts with birth and ends with the engagement in married life. In childhood, Rasas are mostly taught by the parents at an unconscious level, through example and by the creation of a nice atmosphere. Before entering married life, the adolescent student must learn to purify the senses and emotions and get a taste of the finer sentiments so that he or she will be able to live the life of a householder with sufficient control and in good taste. During adolescence, the Rasas are at their peak, so Rasa Yoga makes a lot of sense. Performing various kinds of Rasa Sadhana for shorter periods is the logical approach, with basic control over the main emotions, especially the less desirable ones, the main objective.

❖ The grihastha period of the married householder requires the further development of Rasa-mastery at a time of life when the strongest attachments must be faced toward wife or husband, children, name, fame, possessions, and responsibilities. Depending on a person's talents and profession, this is the stage of Rasa Yoga in which sadhana is performed over longer periods, with the prime objective of excelling in the desirable rajasic Rasas that best support one's role in society and enhance the spiritual path that one may already have taken.

❖ The vanaprastha period starts when the first grandchild is born. This is the time to engage in lifelong Rasa Sadhanas that completely abolish the less desirable Rasas and increase mastery of the most subtle and spiritual Rasas for their own sakes.

❖ When the sanyasa stage of the renunciate starts, the most sattvic Rasas of Calmness, innocent Joy, Devotion, and Compassion become the main objective and even cease to be objectives at all when the highest states of consciousness are attained.

Yoga and Rasas

When performed correctly, all traditional yoga practices are helpful in Rasa Sadhana. Essentially the yogi will choose according to his or her temperament to follow one of the three main yoga paths, each of which, individually or in combination, may lead the yogi to obtaining the union between individual and cosmic consciousness. Each path concentrates on a particular Rasa:

❖ Bhakti Yoga, the path of pure spiritual devotion: focus on Love
❖ Karma Yoga, the path of selfless action: focus on Compassion
❖ Jnana Yoga, the path of right knowledge: focus on Wonder

Courage is essential for any kind of yoga or sadhana, while Joy is the obvious result.

Most schools of yoga follow the eight-fold path of Ashtanga Yoga, in which eight steps must be mastered one after the other, while at the same time remaining as eight limbs of the same tree that all together lead to the final goal. For example, *asana* (posture) prepares the ground for practicing pranayama (breath control), while it also remains essential up to the stage of samadhi.

Asanas are partially designed for the purpose of releasing stress that has been building up in joints, tissues, and organs. For example, they can be used to relieve tensions in the neck region that reduce the blood flow to the brain and increase tamasic Rasas. Emotional blockages are often sustained by physical tensions that can be released through the practice of asanas. Many asanas are simply very relaxing and can be extremely useful when Calmness is used as a pivot between Rasas. Some asanas particularly promote self-confidence, such as the Veeryabhadra Asana. To practice any real meditation, we need at least one posture in which we can be perfectly comfortable for a long time.

Pranayama breathing techniques remove anxiety and depression through the power of prana. Just by slowing down the breathing rate, which is not really pranayama, the Calmness Rasa is invited into our mind. In pranayama, breath suspension *(kumbhaka)* plays a major role and the use of blocks *(bandhas)* allows us to direct the vital force of prana toward the Sushumna Nadi. This yogic breathing may bring out deeply buried emotions from the subconscious and transports us to higher states of consciousness. Alternate nostril breathing balances emotional and rational thought.

Pratyahara, or the withdrawal of sensory perception, purifies the senses and cures us from the pressing desires that are the cause of most emotional disturbances. This subject has already been discussed more generally in chapter 16. The one who has mastered pratyahara has acquired an infallible tool for solving any emotional problem.

The practice of *dharana* or concentration focuses the entire being on the Divine, with the help of sound (mantras, chakra sounds, inner sounds), visualization (deities, yantras, chakras) and concepts (God, the Self, the higher Rasas, the spiritual heart). Reciting mantras is a form of auto-suggestion in the sense that by saying the mantra we also hear it, through the ears or internally. The rhythmic cycle of the mantra directly affects the emotions. All visualization techniques feed the emotional brain hemisphere with subtle energies.

After prolonged practice one can finally reach the stages of *dhyana* (uninterrupted meditation) and *samadhi* (uninterrupted dhyana). Real samadhi takes one completely beyond any emotional problems, because the effect never goes.

Rasas in Yoga Teaching

It is often overlooked that Ashtanga Yoga does not start with the practices of asana, pranayama, pratyahara, and so on. *Yama* (control) and *niyama* (rules of conduct) come first. They represent a set of practical, moral, and spiritual do's and don'ts that prepare the yoga practitioner for successful application of the better-known yoga techniques. Yama includes bodily purity, non-violence, truth, honesty, sexual continence, forbearance, fortitude, kindness, straightforwardness, and moderation in diet. Niyama consists of austerity, contentment, belief in God, charity, worship, study of scriptures, modesty, development of a discerning mind, repetition of prayers, observance of vows, and performance of sacrifices. The practices of yama and niyama are aimed at creating balance in the life of the aspirant. They help in purifying the senses, achieving higher control, and stopping the inner dialogue. They may also include various kinds of fasts, such as food fasts, sleep fasts, speech fasts, sex fasts, and so on.

Without sufficiently sattvic emotions, attempting to follow yama and niyama and seeking higher states of consciousness may be premature. One minute of Anger can destroy much of the balance attained through any kind of yogic exercises. To attain yama and niyama, Rasa Sadhana of various Rasas can be of great help, like Sadhana of Anger (non-violence, forbearance), Courage (fortitude, straightforwardness, austerity, modesty), Compassion (kindness, charity), and so on.

In traditional yoga schools and ashrams, yama and niyama are taught by the entire community and strict disciplines like celibacy have to be followed in order to qualify for real yogic practice. In the West, one becomes "qualified" by simply joining a yoga class. Yoga teachers who have many householders among their students do not have much control over their lives or their practice of yama and niyama. Providing students with Rasa Sadhana exercises to be performed in their daily lives can be a great way to enhance the levels of yama and niyama, enabling the students to obtain far better results in their practice of asana, pranayama, and more advanced yoga techniques. Meditation will naturally deepen and devotion will come more easily. The bottom line is that through Rasa

Sadhana, yoga teachers can help their students to become much happier, thus fulfilling one of the main reasons many people practice yoga.

Teaching Rasa Sadhana is relatively simple. Any yoga teacher can start teaching it after reading this book and trying out these sadhanas on himself or herself. Yoga teachers can be expected to have achieved a relatively good emotional balance in advance, so the shorter sadhanas should be fairly easy for them to master. Their students will first of all need background information on what Rasas really are and how they relate to our body, mind, and so on. In addition, students need basic understanding of the nine different Rasas, how they can be reduced or strengthened, and how sadhana on or from them is to be performed. Teachers can regularly organize evaluation sessions, where people tell of the experiences and problems they have faced with Rasa Sadhana and the teacher can offer more advice and deeper spiritual insights.

Religion and Spirituality

Religion and spiritual practice are more or less organized forms of Bhakti Yoga, the yoga of devotion. In Hindu scriptures, one can see a gradual evolution from the highly theoretical and mystic Vedic knowledge, to a more practical approach in the Brahmanas, Aranyakas, and Upanishads. From all these and later scriptures, the current religious Hindu practices were developed. One might say that religious practices are a form of less conscious yoga created for the masses, but that would give them a less profound character than they merit.

When a religious festival or ceremony is created, positive emotional energy from all parts of the locality or country is brought together. With all attending people thinking of the same thing, vibrating in the same way, an extremely powerful atmosphere is created, first of all on the emotional level. Everybody attending these rituals can be inspired to go into the higher emotional frequencies or Rasas of Love (as devotion), Wonder, Compassion, and Calmness, and take them home afterward. Regular rituals have a profound purifying effect on the spirituality of a community and help it to develop yama and niyama.

Because of its ritualistic nature, religion has a tendency toward stagnation on the intellectual level. Getting stuck in particular views, concepts, and habits is one of the problems caused by the intellect of the individual and this tendency can be further exacerbated by group dynamics. The great asset and power of identification with a group of people of like spiritual attitudes becomes a danger when the ego takes the game a little further into claiming its spiritual path as the only available option. Fundamentalism is not a problem of people sticking firmly to the fundaments of their religion, a common misinterpretation. Fundamentalism enters when people try to force the fundaments of their religion on others. It becomes even more of a problem when such religious groups enter the realm of politics, the struggle for power over the minds and possessions of people.

As we are all different, every individual must follow his or her own path to the Divine, so freedom is a requirement. Hinduism is remarkable because it allows its followers quite absolute freedom. A visitor to India can easily test this by asking all the Hindu people one meets to name their favorite deities. Many diverse answers will be given, with Ganesha, Shiva, Hanuman, Durga, Lakshmi, and many others named. If one then asks the same people about the relationship between their favorite deity and the other Hindu deities, they will all give a similar answer: "Well of course, all Hindu deities are the same god or divine energy, beyond name and form, but I find it easiest to communicate with God in this particular form." The remarkable religious tolerance embedded within the pantheon of countless Hindu deities allows people to experience the Divine in the way that suits them best. This also explains how it is possible for many different deities to be worshipped by members of one and the same Hindu family. Hinduism even has an atheist branch, which is quite accepted by other branches.

Hinduism is also remarkable in its lack of structure and hierarchy in comparison to the other world religions such as Christianity, the Muslim religion, or even Buddhism. Anyone can build a Hindu temple. Anyone can start the worship of a river, tree, mountain, or new idol. Anyone can start preaching and create a religious order. Anyone can invent a new kind of yoga. Hinduism has plenty of tradition and belief in the value of maintaining tradition, as well as sometimes quite strict structures within its religious orders. But it manages at the same time to accept innovation just as well.

In any religion, Hinduism included, the local religious practices may not feel suitable to one's own spiritual approach. And any local religious practice may feel very suitable to one's spiritual needs. Whatever feels good can be good. Religion is about experiencing the Love and Beauty of the Shringara Rasa on a more spiritual level and this can often have a lot more power when done with others rather than alone.

23

Power to the Artists

Modern or traditional, abstract or figurative,
true art is immensely valuable.

Two Branches of Rasa Knowledge

The deepest studies of Rasas have probably been done by actors and other traditional Indian artists. Hindus consider life itself as a divine theatre, so to a Hindu, the actor certainly is seen as a trustworthy and experienced source of knowledge in this matter. In India, the artist is first and foremost someone who understands the art of creating agreeable Rasas in others.

Indian artists who come upon this book might find its knowledge and interpretation of the Rasas quite different from their own. That is because the branch of Rasa Sadhana has its own objectives and hence its own way to interpret and handle the subject. In many ways, the approach in Rasa Sadhana is much more psychological.

To give readers who are less familiar with Indian art a taste of the depth with which Indian art studies the Rasas, following is an overview of the various aspects of the Hasya (Joy) Rasa:

MAIN ASPECTS OF THE HASYA RASA IN INDIAN ART

Rasa (sentiment)	Joy
Bhava (emotion)	Laughter
Varieties	Gentle smile, slight laughter, open laughter, laughter of ridicule, obscene laughter, boisterous laughter
Vibhavas ("determinants": objective conditions that produce the Rasa)	Unseemly dress, misplaced ornaments, impudence, covetousness, quarrel, near-obscene utterance, displaying of deformed limbs, pointing out the faults of others
Anubhavas ("consequents": symptoms of the Rasa produced in the spectator)	Biting the lips, throbbing of the nose and the cheek, opening the eyes wide, contracting the eyes, perspiration, color of the face, holding the sides
Vyabhicari bhavas ("transitory states": states that temporarily occur along with a Rasa, but do not belong to it)	Lethargy, dissimulation, drowsiness, sleeplessness, dreaming, waking up, envy
Types	Atmastha (self based) and Parastha (based in others)

In Indian art the nine Rasas are also expressed by detailed body postures, eye movements, and hand mudras. Anybody who chooses to undertake an in-depth study of the subject of Rasas will find an enormous amount of knowledge in Indian art, which can also be applied to life itself.

Rasa and Bhava

For the sake of simplicity little distinction between emotion and sentiment has been made in this book, as it is of little value in Rasa Sadhana. In Indian art, however, there are important differences between Rasa as sentiment and Bhava as mood or emotion.

On a literal level, Rasa is "that which is being enjoyed (tasted)." Bhava means "that which becomes." Bhava becomes Rasa as the finer sentiment is generated by the emotion: The Bhava expressed by the artist induces the Rasa in the spectator or connoisseur *(rasika)*. Artistic creation is the distillation of a Bhava as Rasa, an essence that is freed from all distinctions in time and space by the creative intuition called *pratibha.* From the point of view of the spectator, what he or she experiences goes beyond the emotional content (Bhava) of the drama or other art form and becomes a clarified essence of emotion (Rasa).

In Indian art Rasa means the awareness that rises above the poetic content, the stage spectacle, the music, and so on and generalizes the emotional states of the spectators into a single emotional "field." As mentioned earlier, in the Natya Shastra* eight Rasas are recognized and related to what are called the eight dominant Bhavas:

RASA AND BHAVA IN INDIAN ART

Bhava	Rasa
Rati (love)	Shringara (erotic)
Hasa (merriment)	Hasya (humorous)
Shoka (sorrow)	Karuna (pathos)
Krodha (fury)	Raudra (anger)
Utsaha (enthusiasm)	Veerya (heroic)
Bhaya (terror)	Bhayanaka (terrifying)
Jugupsa (disgust)	Vibhatsa (odious)
Vismaya (astonishment)	Adbhuta (mysterious)

Rasas, Ragas, and Dance

Four elements are essential in classical Indian music, both in north as in south India:

---

*Bharatamuni, *The Natya Sastra* (Delhi: Sri Satguru Publications, 2000).

❖ *Raga*: scale/melody
❖ *Rasa*: sentiment
❖ *Bhava*: mood
❖ *Tala*: rhythm

Each raga is dominated by one Rasa, even if the performer can also produce other sentiments in a less prominent way. The more the notes of a raga conform to a single emotion, the more overwhelming the effect of the raga.

Some principal notes were associated with specific Rasas by Bharata:

RASAS EXPRESSED AS MUSICAL NOTES

Rasa	Indian Notes	Corresponding Western Notes
Shringara, Hasya	Ma, Pa	Fa, Sol
Veerya, Raudra, Adbhuta	Sa, Ri	Do, Re
Karuna	Ga, Ni	Mi, Ti
Vibhatsa, Bhayanaka	Dha	La

These are used as principal notes in compositions that are designed to create specific Rasas. It is not only the single notes that affect the Rasa, but also their combination in melody and rhythm. Not all ragas are designed to stimulate one Rasa. Some are created for a special occasion, season, or time of the day; they may have a dominant Rasa, but most often create a sequence of Rasas.

Rasas also play a dominant role in classical Indian dance. Bharata Natyam is one of the main classical dance styles in India, developed from ritualistic dances performed in temples and at the ancient courts. Bharata Natyam is an artistic yoga (Natya Yoga), a way of revealing the spiritual through the corporeal. Its name partially refers to saint Bharata who wrote the Natya Shastra, the standard classical volume on Rasas. Shringara is seen as the supreme emotion that reflects the mystic union of the human with the Divine. Bharata Natyam is a means of spiritual elevation both for the dancer and the audience. The jewelry worn by the dancer stimulates the chakras and balances lunar and solar energies. Other dance styles pay equal importance to the Rasas, such as the Kathakali, Kuchipudi, Manipuri, Orissi, and Kathak dance traditions.

Objectives of Indian Art

The central objective of classical Indian art is to create Rasas in the spectators, in order to communicate or suggest a kind of knowledge that cannot be clearly expressed in words. The knowledge of Rasas is not revealed or explained (as it is in this book), but manifested inside the spectator, which makes it very powerful, leading to real knowledge of truth through intuitive understanding. Thus art becomes a means for educating and healing people emotionally. Even when the intuitive insight does not continue, the truth one has realized remains as faith.

Art is a very precise expression of philosophy and, in India, philosophy has been expressed in a very artistic way. The ancient scriptures such as the Vedas, Puranas, and Upanishads were written as beautiful verses by rishis, saints, seers, and visionaries who were also poets. All spirituality that is known to the world does not come from God, because God is beyond language. But God provides the inspiration. Inspiration can only come to people who are in tune with the Divine. Those who are depressed, those who are only thinking about their future, their social status, name, and fame can never create really valuable art. Only pure beings create pure art. Through the application of Rasa Sadhana to his or her own life, an artist may master all of the Rasas, and thus purify his or her aesthetic sense to such a degree that the art produced also becomes pure. Thus the greatest artist is a saint who contemplates, concentrates, meditates, and creates symbols that can really touch the spectator. That is why true art and spirituality are inseparable.

For the Indian artist, the main objective is not the expression of personal feelings. Creating art is an act of worship, a meditative process that brings the artist closer to the Divine. Traditional Indian arts always portrayed religious feelings, which lifted people into a higher sphere of life. All spirituality and philosophy needs expression. It needs to be drawn, painted, sculptured, danced, and played so that it leaves a deep impression in the spectators who can then try to live accordingly.

Rules in Indian Art

All branches of Indian art have their own rules, but with regard to the Rasas they all more or less stick to the same point of view. In order to meet the objective of creating Rasas in the spectators and transferring spiritual or philosophical knowledge through them, classical Indian art will try to cover all Rasas found in life, but will focus on the most desirable Rasas.

Most of the time, a poem, a work of literature, or a painting will be focused on one Rasa only. But that main or *sthayi* Rasa will also have supportive or *sancarin* Rasas. Shringara is most often the main Rasa, accompanied by Courage, Joy, and Wonder. Anger, Fear, Sadness, and especially Disgust are to be used sparingly.

Less agreeable Rasas may also enter Indian art, but mostly to create the contrast that makes the agreeable Rasas even more powerful. If the hero is not faced with something terrifying, then it is more difficult to demonstrate his Courage. The person of good taste becomes even more an expression of Shringara if contrasted with a vulgar person. Even though in ancient Indian plays, the end always had to be good and uplifting, during the drama Sadness often played an important role.

Due to their personal temperament, many artists are only capable of creating art that produces one or a few Rasas. When an artist can integrate all nine Rasas in proper proportion he or she becomes a master. A poem that includes all nine Rasas becomes a *mahakavya*, a "great" poem.

Modern Art

Using new ways to create art, new media, and new techniques is fantastic. In order to remain interested, both spectators and artists need variation. Abstract art can be just as effective in evoking Rasas as other art, as is also demonstrated by the ancient use of yantras (geometrical patterns). Novelty in art is fine as long as it does not become the main objective, the message getting lost in self-centered obscurity.

Art is an expression that has to be informed by the time, the age, and the problems of the age. In very early times, Wonder and Love in the form of devotion to the Divine were the main Rasas in art, which mostly served ritual. When society developed and kings came, then Love, Joy, and Courage became important subjects. When dharma in Love, Joy, and Courage was lost (the period of the Mahabharata), Sadness became a topic.

In modern times, the artist gives an expression of how society has gone away from wholeness. Naturally, less agreeable Rasas such as Fear, Anger, and Disgust have become more dominant in modern art. Those artists who understand that they are messengers and reformers know that there is a relation between their conduct and their art. They know that if they live as pure beings their art will be pure. And they also know that by creating art with pure and desirable Rasas, their own Rasas and life will benefit from it. Even if these times require them to include less desirable Rasas in their art, when they include them in proper proportion, so that the main feeling created is still enjoyable, they can enjoy it also.

Unfortunately many artists are so absorbed by the less desirable Rasas that they create art purely out of Anger, Disgust, Sadness, and Fear. The expression gives them some kind of satisfaction and such art may also naturally attract attention because it is seen as innovative (Adbhuta) and courageous (Veerya). In this way these artists become trapped by their success and ego. In order to satisfy their public, they always need to find new ways to be remarkable by delving deeper into their darkest emotions, which makes them suffer personally.

If the art only communicates problems and offers no solutions, then the public also will suffer from it and the art will only enhance the more demonic feelings in society. Such art is of bad taste and very unhealthy, both for the artist and for the spectators. Whether the artist is talented and skilled or not makes no difference.

There have been times when the ruling classes have censured art in order to hide the disagreeable Rasas that were the result of their twisted policies. Today, we are all too aware of the demonic side of life, so while it needs no hiding, it also requires no promotion.

If an artist can remain sincere in his or her work, then it is still art. If the artist becomes trapped by his or her ego and the negative emotions being expressed, then art becomes an expression of mental disease, perhaps suitable as a therapeutic activity for the artist, but unsuitable for bringing truth to society. If artists feel the need to express the problems of these modern times, then that need must include the desire to contribute to solutions, otherwise it is insincere, demonic, ego-centered, sick, or simply greedy.

To sum up, there is nothing wrong with including the less desirable Rasas in art, as long as the whole remains uplifting. Whether it is a painting, a song, a movie, or a poem, the main objective of art must be spiritual or philosophical, an expression of divine values, ideas, and feelings. Such art and the artists that create it are of high importance to society. Using great works of art in the decoration of our homes and cities can be a powerful way of cultivating the desirable Rasas.

24

Social Work and Politics

*While poverty may be an excuse for feeling bad,
many do not need it.*

Rasas and Castes

In the Indian Rasa tradition, particular Rasas were attributed to particular castes *(varnas)*. This was not originally intended in the way that it was sometimes interpreted later, when agreeable Rasas were seen as the prerogative of the higher castes and the less agreeable Rasas as the fate of the lower castes. The original intent was to show the relationship between social status and the dominating quality of the Rasas that may result from it.

DOMINATING RASAS IN THE VARNAS

Varna	Caste	Dominating Rasas
Brahmin	Priests	Love, Joy, Wonder, Calmness
Kshatriya	Warriors	Anger, Courage
Vaishya	Merchants	Sadness
Shudra	Servants	Fear, Disgust

Those who are concerned about the quality of Rasas in society cannot ignore the impact of social status. If one often has difficulty in making ends meet, like a Shudra, then Fear and Disgust are hard to avoid. If one is often caught by Fear and Disgust, then one's actions more easily become disgusting and terrifying to others, whether one is a Shudra or a Brahmin. While it is principally unjust, this interaction explains why higher castes and especially Brahmins began to look upon the lowest castes as untouchable, fearsome, and disgusting.

The life of a Brahmin is the most suitable to develop the agreeable Rasas, because a Brahmin lives on minimum requirements but rests assured of access to basic needs. The practice of disciplines and the concentration on dharma, devotion, and truth also helps.

The Anger Rasa is most suitable to the warrior caste, as Anger can be a useful tool for people who must defend their own. Anger is friendly to the more agreeable Courage Rasa that is the main Rasa attributed to this caste.

A merchant is often too busy to develop and enjoy Calmness, Love and Beauty, Wonder, or Joy and Humor. And he has too much to lose to become a hero or a warrior. He is expected to be kind to every customer, may feel pity for others who are less assured of wealth, and may distribute some of his own wealth in charity. Hence Karuna is the dominating Rasa.

Rasas and Social Work

The above demonstrates two principles that are actually very common knowledge in any culture: Money doesn't make you happy but having no money is not a good option either if your stomach is empty. For those who are interested in social work, it means first of all that the basic material needs of people must be met. But it also means that to help those people be happy when their basic material needs are met, it is more efficient to concentrate on spreading truth and the agreeable Rasas than to continue increasing their wealth.

Social work should thus combine basic material help with the promotion of spiritual knowledge, art, joy, and so on. All desires are ultimately desires for happiness, so if people can be taught to pursue happiness more directly, it will be the very best help one can provide. One cannot blame poorer people who desire the security and pleasures of wealth that they see in others, but one does not need to help them in pursuing those illusions.

Rasas and Politics

In ancient India, politics were the task of the kings who belonged to the warrior caste. When the country was attacked, they were responsible for defending it. When the country was at peace they needed to have equal courage and determination in ruling it to the benefit of their people.

In modern times, the question is: "What benefits the people?" Politicians should structure society in such a way that it takes care of the basic needs of everybody and spend whatever resources remain on promoting the more agreeable Rasas through art, enjoyment, and education. Unfortunately, politicians with the Courage required to take care of both are few. Most politicians are so absorbed in the worship of the deity of wealth—which they call Economy—that they do not even care. They do not respect dharma in their power struggles, but abuse the less agreeable Rasas of the people to gain worldly power by deceit and faulty rhetoric.

One can easily understand the importance given by the Vishnu Purana (see chapter 20) to the greed of the rulers in causing the loss of morality in general. Rulers and the ruling classes have so often abused morality for their own gain that it is not surprising to see so many people losing belief in moral values and regarding anyone claiming them as hypocritical. Religious leaders entering the power struggle have not exactly been very helpful in changing that dynamic; in fact the opposite has often been true.

These abuses are just another sorry aspect of this Kali Yuga age, which one day will pass. Kings come and go, and so do presidents, prime ministers, and political parties. If one wishes to pursue the agreeable Rasas, then entering politics is not an easy road. In a war fought by unfair means, it is difficult not to become tainted. It is only an option for those who feel they have the Courage needed to fight for justice without violence in thought, word, or deed.

25

Mood Marketing

*Whatever happiness advertising promises,
we already have at our disposal.*

Rasas in Marketing

Advertising specialists know very well that the desire to purchase a product is often more strongly influenced by unconscious emotional attraction than by conscious rational evaluation. In marketing seminars, this is often symbolized by the partially submerged iceberg of buying values:

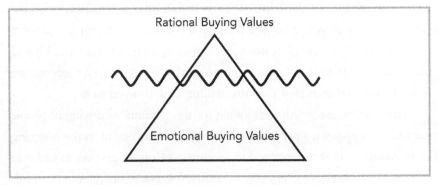

Figure 25.1. Rational and Emotional Buying Values.

The rational values upon which purchases are based may be seen above the water: They are easily apparent to consumers, salespeople, and marketers. They mostly consist of practical needs and desires. The most important part of the iceberg, however, remains largely invisible; it consists of emotional values such as prestige, security, enjoyment, curiosity, and so on. Salespeople and marketers are taught to stimulate these values through the use of emotionally loaded words, images, shop atmosphere, and so on. Consumers then start buying products without practical need, because they unconsciously expect these products to provide them with the emotional states that they desire: To make them feel beautiful, rich, secure, powerful, and so on.

Most consumers obviously have some idea of this process, but very few realize that the power of advertising goes far beyond any normal level of emotional control. It is easily demonstrated that the use of desirable sights, sounds, and even smells (in supermarkets for example) can be used to change people's biochemistry in such a way that it makes them dissatisfied and more eager to buy.

Advertising makes people unhappy and drives this world crazy. It shows us more beautiful women and men in just one day than we are likely to meet in real life during an entire lifetime. While feminists rightfully complain about many ads being degrading to women, nobody seems to wonder about what these ads do to men.

While art produces pleasure by depicting the lives of characters who have more drama in their lives than is usual, advertising produces dissatisfaction by showing people with perfect lives. Advertising and most popular entertainment continuously impose upon us levels of wealth and material security that only the richest can afford. Moreover, there are no limits to the methods that they are willing and allowed to use.

The only excuse worth mentioning for this continuous driving of people toward unhappiness, a permanent sense of non-fulfillment, is the boosting of an economy that is perceived to require continuous growth in order to meet the basic needs of everyone. In reality, it keeps many people from fulfilling those basic needs, by making others so addicted to buying and consumption that they mindlessly devour much more than they really need.

People who wish to keep their Rasas pure must avoid advertising and most of modern entertainment as well, as already explained in chapter 16. Every ad could be met with the prayer "Please leave my biochemistry in peace," if it merits even that much attention.

Mood Products

As science has recently brought the body-mind link to the attention of society, one might hope that it could lead society to put more limits on advertising and commerce. That would not be easy, but quite necessary, especially in the light of what follows.

The main result of the growing consciousness about the body-mind link is that products are now slowly being promoted more directly in relation to their emotional effects. This happens through the adaptation of the advertising for existing products (such as sugar, chocolate, vitamins, meat, and coffee), as well as through the creation of new products, so called "mood products," that may contain high doses of vitamins, minerals, and many stimulating, relaxing, or euphoria-inducing ingredients such as ayahuasca, colanut, damiana, datura, ephedrine, guarana, kava kava, ketamine, and khat. While most of these adaptations in marketing are still rather tentative and fairly innocent, it can be predicted that soon toothpastes will "wake you up," fabrics will "massage your skin" and steaks will "help you through the day." This is not necessarily a bad turn of events, but is dangerous nevertheless.

Many mood foods and other so-called mood enhancing products are often based on the faulty interpretation of incomplete scientific facts, as explained in chapter 21. That makes them have no value and they might even cause adverse effects. Even more importantly, these products give people the idea that happiness can be bought. They thus reinforce a culture of purposeless zipping from one kick to another. The stronger these mood products become, the more they contribute to the creation of a culture of drug addiction (see chapter 3). The use of antidepressants, calming agents, and stimulating agents is already extremely high in Western society, even though it is often legally limited to prescription by doctors. For example, in Belgium—a European country with less than ten million inhabitants—over fourteen million packages of sleep-inducing and calming agents, 5.7 million packages of anti-depressants, and 300,000 packages of stimulants (not including Viagra) were sold in the year 2000, according to the Ministry of Health.

Less powerful mood products easily escape legal prescription, leaving the doors wide open for abuse. They are likely to cause far more devastating if less obvious effects than those produced by illegal drugs. As explained in chapter 3, there is nothing wrong with mildly directing one's Rasas through the senses, food, spices, and so on. Products that are designed to alter moods (as all products are, even without their makers being conscious of it) should be equally mild. Using products that dramatically alter one's moods literally destroys one's self-confidence and natural ability for happiness.

26

Rasas in Therapy

No doctor can cure disease all by himself.

Some people have psychological problems whose origin and therapeutic cure goes far beyond the Rasas and the scope of this book. They have often suffered from extreme emotional states that have damaged their intellect and require very special help and healing.

The problems of most people who visit therapists are, however, largely emotional. These people are so caught by imaginary Fear, uncontrollable Anger, inconsolable Sadness, or self-destructive Disgust that they feel in need of help to get free. They are victims of the poor quality of Rasas and morality in society and of their own ignorance about their emotional nature and the nature of truth.

The information on Rasas given in this book thus can be of great help to therapists. Rasa Sadhana can be a powerful tool in the recovery process of patients who suffer from sleep disturbances, addictions, relational problems, worries, depression, and so on. It may need to be adapted to the patient's level of self-control, by making the rules less strict. If even one day without Anger is too much, then one hour may be a good start.

In Ayurveda, a therapist is primarily regarded as a teacher. Analysis and counseling may be part of the job, but teaching the ways to reach balance in body and mind is the main task. The Ayurvedic therapist may use certain therapies that are relaxing, detoxifying, energizing, and so on in order to help the patient to achieve that balance. But when the way to maintain balance is not also taught, the therapies only assure the therapist of a stable stream of patients.

Many people who seek out therapists would be better helped by *satsang*, keeping the company of saints and gurus. A guru is the one who leads us from darkness to light, from ignorance to truth. Those who feel enveloped by darkness should seek this light.

One of the problems in modern society is that most information on emotional issues originates from the study and treatment of people with exceptional emotional blockages. It often causes relatively "normal" people to think that they must have similar blockages that require special treatment and even medication. However, most people are perfectly capable of changing their emotional patterns without any need for those desperate measures, provided they believe that they have that power.

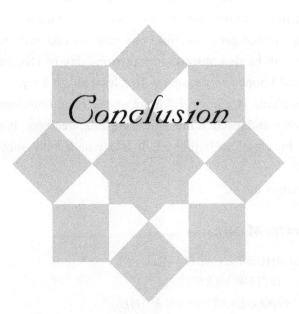

Conclusion

One of the working titles for this book was *Tabula Rasa,* an ancient Latin saying that literally means "to start with a new, clean, wax tablet or *tabula.*" The title was not easy to understand without this explanation, so it was not used. Still, the message that it includes is essential. When we start to understand what our Rasas really are, we should come to the conclusion that it is time to stop wasting our happiness in disagreeable moods and choose a fresh start.

Feeling good or bad is a matter of choice. Whatever unpleasant thing happens is only unpleasant if we let our Rasas follow it. When something does not function as it should, or somebody does something bad, or we ourselves do something stupid: If we let such things make us feel bad, then we make ourselves suffer so much more. To stop this silly game becomes common sense.

Through this understanding we reduce all our problems to a single question: "How can we achieve control over our Rasas?" Regular exercise through Rasa Sadhana is the answer, supported by a spiritual approach to life, healthy cooking, balancing sensory input, and maintaining rather simple daily routines that keep us in tune with nature. It takes a while to develop the right reactions, to create and strengthen the correct neural patterns, to achieve the required level of balance in our body chemistry. And without true exercise, it will take a lot longer. But step-by-step we can get there and every step we take will make us feel better. This can be demonstrated by just one day of Disgust or Anger Sadhana, and I hope every reader will at least give it a try.

Rasa Sadhana is a powerful Yoga of the Nine Emotions that anybody can learn and teach. It may not bring enlightenment, but will bring us quite a bit closer to happiness. It is a wonderfully simple kind of magic.

Please enjoy it.

GAYATRI MANTRA

AUM BHUR BHUVAH SVAH
TAT SAVITUR VARENYAM
BHARGO DEVASYA DHI MAHI
DHIYO YO NAH PRACHODAYAT

Almighty God who pervades all planes
Who is the most bright and exalted
Devoid of sin and divine
Inspire our intellect to follow the righteous path of meditation.

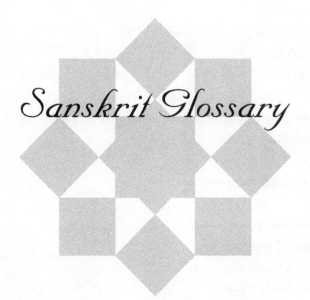

Sanskrit Glossary

Adbhuta – Wonder, mystery

ahamkara – I-consciousness, ego

ahimsa – non-violence

ahladini shakti – the energy of joy

akasha – the element of space, void, ether

ananda – bliss

anandamaya kosha – sheath of Self or bliss

anima – boundlessness

anna – food

annamaya kosha – sheath of matter

apana – one of the five main pranas

apsara – celestial dancing maiden

asana – posture

Ashtanga Yoga – the classical eight-fold path of yoga

Ayurveda – ancient Indian science of life for physical and mental well-being

bandha – yogic lock

bhakti – devotion, divine love

bhava – emotion
Bhayanaka – Fear, terror
bhukti - enjoyment
bodhisattva – a compassionate one
Brahmin - priestly caste
buddhi – intellect

chakras – seven energy centers, each associated with a particular state of
   consciousness
chit – truth
chitta – being, the feeling self

deva – divine being
Devi – (mother) goddess
dharana – concentration
dharma – code of conduct
dhatus – seven constituents of the human body
dhyana – meditation
doshas – humors, temperaments

gandharva – celestial musician
gopi – milk maiden
gunas – qualities of energy
guru – spiritual guide

Hasya – Joy, Humor

ichcha - omnipotence
ida – lunar nadi
ishatattva – the power to rule

japa – repetition (of mantra)
jiva – the individual self
jivan – life
jnana – knowledge (gyana)

Kali Yuga – age of iron and conflict

kama – enjoyment

Kama Sutra – scripture on (sensual) enjoyment

kapha – the dosha formed by water and earth

karma – law of cause and effect

Karuna – compassion, pity, Sadness

kosha – sheath

Kshatriya – warrior caste

kumbhaka – breath suspension

kundalini – the spiritual energy that lies dormant at the base of the spine until awakened

laghima – lightness

leela – sport, play, game

lingam – male generative organ

loka – plane

mahima – mightiness

manas – mind

manomaya kosha – sheath of mind

mantra – sacred formula/praise/request addressed to a specific deity

mantra japa – mantra repetition

marmas – pressure points

maya – illusion, the veiling power of existence

moksha – liberation

mudra – a muscular control practice that aids meditation; hand posture; expression of emotional state by control of facial, limbic, and bodily muscles

nadi – carrier of subtle energy in the body

niyama – rules of conduct in yoga

ojas – primary vigor, personal magnetism

pingala – solar nadi

pitta – the dosha formed by fire and water

prakam – power to assume any form

prakriti – primordial nature

prana – vital life force

pranamaya kosha – sheath of vital air

pranayama – conscious breath control

prapti – attainment

pratibha – creative intuition

pratyahara – sense withdrawal

puja (pooja) – worship, ritual

purusha – primordial soul, creative consciousness

raga – scale, melody

rajas – passion, activity, mobility

rakshasa - demon

Rasa – essence of emotion, taste, mood

Rasa Vidya – science of alchemy

rasayana – rejuvenating agents

Raudra – Anger

rishi – seer or saint

sadhana – practice, exercise

samadhi – realized nonduality, complete balance

sambhoga shringara – feeling love in union

Sanskrit – ancient language of India

sat – truth *(satya)*

sati – widow burning

satsang – the company of saints

sattva – equanimity, lightness, purity

shakti – energized consciousness, goddess

Shanta – Calmness, peace

shastra – scripture

Shringara – Love, beauty, adoration

Shudra – servant caste

siddhi – power, accomplishment, attainment

soma – nectar, lunar principle

sushumna – the main nadi that passes through the spinal column

Swar Yoga – a yoga based on the science of breath

tala – rhythm

tamas – sloth, inertia, darkness

tanmatra – pure essence, frequency, principle

tantra – expanded consciousness

tapasya – austerity, penance

tattva – element

tejas – the inner radiance, the fierce principle

Vaishya – merchant caste

vashitva – popularity

vastu – art of harmony at home

vata – the dosha formed by air and akasha

vatsalya rasa – rasa of parental love

vayu – air

vedic – of the vedas, sacred teachings

Veerya – Courage, self-confidence

Vibhatsa – Disgust, dissatisfaction

vidya – knowledge

vijnanamaya kosha – sheath of ego and intellect

vipaka – power of foods after digestion

vipralambha shringara – feeling of love in separation, longing

virya – power of foods during digestion

vrittis – mental modifications

yantra – shape, form, pattern

Yama – control; the lord of death

yoga – to unite, join

yogi – practitioner of yoga

References and Recommended Reading

Annapoorna, L., ed. *New Dimensions of Indian Music, Dance and Drama.* New Delhi: Sundeep Prakashan, 1998.

Bharatamuni. *The Natya Sastra.* Delhi: Sri Satguru Publications, 2000.

Bhattacharya, Narendra. *History of the Tantric Religion.* New Delhi: Manohar Publishers, 1999.

Chand, Devi. *The Atharvaveda* (Sanskrit text with English translation). New Delhi: Munshiram Manoharlal Publishers, 1999.

Council of Scientific and Industrial Research. *The Wealth of India.* New Delhi: Council of Scientific and Industrial Research, 1985.

Damasio, Antonio. *The Feeling of What Happens.* New York: Harcourt, Brace & Company, 1999.

Dash, Bhagwan, and Lalitesh Kashyap. *Rasa Sastra, Iatro-chemistry of Ayurveda.* New Delhi: Concept Publishing Company, 1994.

Eldershaw, Jane. *Mood Food: Brighten, Heal, and Elevate Your State of Mind.* Naperville, Ill.: Sourcebooks, Inc., 2001.

Ellis, Hattie. *Mood Food: Strategies for Contemporary Cooking and Entertaining.* London: Trafalgar Square Publishing, 1998.

Frawley, David. *Ayurveda and the Mind*. Delhi: Lotus Press, 2000.

———. *Yoga and Ayurveda*. Twin Lakes, Wis.: Lotus Press, 1999.

Gautam, M. R. *Evolution of Raga and Tala in Indian Music*. New Delhi: Munshiram Manoharlal Publishers, 1993.

Gnoli, Raniero. *The Aesthetic Experience According to Abhinavagupta*. Varanasi: Chowkhamba Sanskrit Series Office, 1985.

Goleman, Daniel. *Emotional Intelligence*. New York: Bantam, 1995.

Greenfield, Susan. *Brain Story*. Baarn, the Netherlands: Bosch & Keuning, 2001.

Griffith, Ralph T. H. *Hymns of the Rig Veda*. New Delhi: Munshiram Manoharlal Publishers, 1987.

Johari, Harish. *Ayurvedic Healing Cuisine: 200 Vegetarian Recipes for Health, Balance, and Longevity*. Rochester, Vt.: Healing Arts Press, 2000.

———. *Ayurvedic Massage*. Rochester, Vt.: Healing Arts Press, 1996.

———. *Breath, Mind, and Consciousness*. Rochester, Vt.: Destiny Books, 1989.

———. *Chakras*. Rochester, Vt.: Destiny Books, 2000.

———. *Dhanwantari*. Rochester, Vt.: Healing Arts Press, 1998.

———. *The Healing Power of Gemstones*. Rochester, Vt.: Destiny Books, 1996.

———. *Leela: The Game of Self-Knowledge*. Rochester, Vt.: Destiny Books, 1993.

———. *Numerology, with Tantra, Ayurveda, and Astrology*. Rochester, Vt.: Destiny Books, 1900.

Kuppuswamy, B. *Elements of Ancient Indian Psychology*. Delhi: Konark Publishers, 1990.

Null, Gary. *The Food-Mood-Body Connection: Nutrition-Based and Environmental Approaches to Mental Health and Physical Well-Being*. New York: Seven Stories Press, 2002.

Null, Gary, and Dr. Martin Feldman. *Good Food, Good Mood*. New York: St. Martin's Press, 2001.

Oschman, James L. *Energy Medicine*. Edinburgh, U.K.: Harcourt Publishers Limited, 2000.

Pert, Candace B. *The Molecules of Emotion*. New York: Scribner, 1997.

Rao, Suvarnalata. *Acoustical Perspective on Raga-Rasa Theory*. New Delhi: Munshiram Manoharlal Publishers, 2000.

Ross, Julia. *The Diet Cure: The 8-Step Program to Rebalance Your Body Chemistry and End Food Cravings, Weight Problems, and Mood Swings*. New York: Penguin, 2000.

Rowell, Lewis. *Music and Musical Thought in Early India*. New Delhi: Munshiram Manoharlal Publishers, 1999.

Sastry, Ananthakrishna. *Lalita Sahasranama*. Chennai: Adyar Library, 1999.

Somer, Elisabeth, and Nancy Snyderman. *Food and Mood: The Complete Guide to Eating Well and Feeling Your Best*. 2nd ed. New York: Owl Books, 1999.

Sharma, S. N. *A History of Vedic Literature*. Varanasi: Chowkhambha Sanskrit Series Office, 2000.

Thayer, Robert. *Calm Energy: How People Regulate Mood with Food and Exercise*. New York: Oxford University Press, 2001.

Vingerhoets, Guy, and Engelien Lannoo. *Handboek Neuropsychologie: de biologische basis van het gedrag*. Amersfoort, the Netherlands: Acco Leuven, 1998.

Wiley, Rudolf. *Biobalance: The Acid/Alkaline Solution to the Food-Mood-Health Puzzle*. Orem, Utah: Essential Science Publishing, 1988.

Wurtman, Judith. *Managing Your Mind and Mood Through Food*. New York: HarperCollins, 1988.

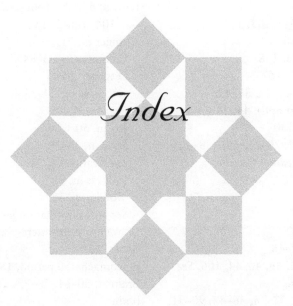

Index

Harish Johari (1934–1999) was a distinguished North Indian author, tantric scholar, poet, musician, composer, artist, and gemologist who held degrees in philosophy and literature and made it his life's work to introduce the spirituality of his homeland to the West. He authored twelve books on a wide range of related subjects, including *Chakras, Tools for Tantra, Ayurvedic Healing Cuisine, Dhanwantari,* and *Leela, the Game of Self-Knowledge.* He also produced meditative audio-recordings, such as *The Sounds of Tantra, The Sounds of the Chakras,* and *Meditation Music for Dawn and Dusk.*

Peter Marchand was born in 1963 in Belgium and studied philosophy, communication sciences, and environmental engineering. Since 1986 he has worked on the development of healthy and environmentally sound products. He became a student of Harish Johari in 1983 and organized the Rasa Sadhana workshop by Harish Johari in 1997. Today he is one of the main founders of the Sanatan Society, a networking organization of family and students of Harish Johari. He travels to India once or twice a year and also teaches Rasa Sadhana.

Visit the author's website for updates and teaching schedules:

www.rasas.info

Visit the Sanatan Society websites for Indian art, free wallpapers, and free information on Hindu deities, yoga, meditation, Indian astrology, Ayurvedic massage, home remedies, vegetarian recipes, online mantras . . .

www.sanatansociety.com

www.sanatansociety.org

BOOKS OF RELATED INTEREST

The Yoga of Truth
Jnana: The Ancient Path of Silent Knowledge
by Peter Marchand

Chakras
Energy Centers of Transformation
by Harish Johari

The Heart of Yoga
Developing a Personal Practice
by T. K. V. Desikachar

Microchakras
Techniques for InnerTuning
by Sri Shyamji Bhatnagar and David Isaacs, Ph.D.

The Yoga-Sūtra of Patañjali
A New Translation and Commentary
by Georg Feuerstein, Ph.D.

Layayoga
The Definitive Guide to the Chakras and Kundalini
by Shyam Sundar Goswami

Chakra Frequencies
Tantra of Sound
by Jonathan Goldman and Andi Goldman

Yoga Spandakarika
The Sacred Texts at the Origins of Tantra
by Daniel Odier

Inner Traditions • Bear & Company
P.O. Box 388
Rochester, VT 05767
1-800-246-8648
www.InnerTraditions.com

Or contact your local bookseller